Overcoming Complications of

LASIK

and Other Eye Surgeries

WITHDRAWN

Ismail A. Shalaby, MD, PhD
Dean A. Haycock, PhD

SUNRISE
River Press

SUNRISE River Press

Sunrise River Press
39966 Grand Avenue
North Branch, MN 55056
Phone: 651-277-1400 or 800-895-4585
Fax: 651-277-1203
www.sunriseriverpress.com

Dedication

For Rafeef

For Marie

Edit by Karin Craig
Layout by Monica Seiberlich

ISBN 978-1-934716-02-1
Item No. SRP602

Library of Congress Cataloging-in-Publication Data

Shalaby, Ismail A.
  Overcoming complications of LASIK and other eye surgeries / by Ismail A. Shalaby and Dean A. Haycock.
       p. cm.
  Includes bibliographical references and index.
  ISBN 978-1-934716-02-1
  1. LASIK (Eye surgery)--Complications. 2. Eye--Surgery--Complications. I. Haycock, Dean A. II. Title.
  RE85.S53 2010
  617.7'190598--dc22

                              2009051547

Printed in USA
10 9 8 7 6 5 4 3 2 1

Table of Contents

Table of Contents *continued*

Preface

Millions of people now enjoy good vision due to the knowledge and skill of ophthalmologists, optometrists, and other eye care professionals. These include the fast-growing number of people who have been pleased with the results of their refractive eye surgery, freeing them from their need for contact lenses or glasses. Every year in the United States, around one million people have some form of laser vision correction surgery. Seventy percent of them "feel amazed and delighted" with the results three months later, according to one survey. For many of the remaining 30 percent, however, the feelings are less positive.

Results of the United States Food and Drug Administration (FDA) studies indicate that six months after eye surgery, more than 20 percent of patients have uncomfortably dry eyes, around 18 percent have glare or halos, and 19 percent have trouble driving after dark. These estimates need to be confirmed by a careful study that accurately determines statistics regarding complications following refractive eye surgery, but they emphasize that the procedures are not for everyone, 100-percent guaranteed or trouble-free.

In response to patient complaints, the FDA is planning a large, national study to examine the relationship of LASIK (laser-assisted *in situ* keratomileusis) complications and quality of life, including psychological problems, such as depression.

Before you undergo any type of eye surgery, it is important to be aware of potential complications before and after surgery. For example, about 20 percent of people who have cataract surgery see very well initially but gradually develop blurred vision months to years after the operation. The most common cause of this impaired vision can be corrected easily in most cases, but it can be disturbing for those affected by it if they aren't informed in advance about the possibility.

Many of the complications described in this book, if they occur, are detected by routine follow-up exams and treated in a routine manner by your doctor. That is why it is important to always follow your doctor's advice and never miss a routine, annual eye examination or a postsurgical follow-up examination.

If, in the statistically unlikely event that you experience a complication following any type of eye surgery, you should be able to recognize the problem and get appropriate care as soon as necessary. In some rare cases, this may mean a visit to an emergency room if your ophthalmologist can't see you immediately. In other cases, it may mean spending time seeking specialists who have experience treating lingering, nonemergency problems such as persistent dry eyes or night-vision problems following refractive eye surgery. This book describes and addresses both types of situations.

Complications, like diseases, often respond best to treatment if they are recognized early. We hope the information provided in this book better equips you to spot trouble as soon as possible in the unlikely event it develops after your eye surgery.

Ismail A. Shalaby, MD, PhD , Dean A. Haycock, PhD

Acknowledgments

Our skilled, patient editor at Sunrise River Press, Karin Craig, suggested the topic of this book. Our friends and families graciously supported us and tolerated our absences as deadlines approached.

About the Authors

Ismail A. Shalaby, MD, PhD, is a board-certified medical and surgical ophthalmologist in private practice and an instructor in ophthalmology at Friedenwald Eye Institute in Baltimore, Maryland. He obtained his PhD in pharmacology and neurosciences at The University of Chicago and his MD from The Johns Hopkins School of Medicine in Baltimore. He has been in solo private practice for ten years. Aside from his active ophthalmology career, Dr. Shalaby is also CEO of Nema Research Inc., a clinical trial implementation company. Dr. Shalaby has authored and coauthored numerous peer-reviewed research articles in pharmacology, drug discovery, neurosciences, and ophthalmology. He has also been a reviewer and on editorial boards of various scientific journals. His latest publication is a chapter on ocular syphilis in a standard reference text of ophthalmology, *Current Ocular Therapy* (sixth edition, 2008). He has lectured and been a past speaker for various pharmaceutical firms.

Dean Haycock, PhD, is a freelance science and medical writer based in New York. He earned a PhD in neuroscience from the department of biology and medicine at Brown University. His research has been published in numerous academic journals including the *Journal of Neurochemistry, Journal of Medicinal Chemistry, Journal of Pharmacology and Experimental Therapeutics,* and *Brain Research.* His past and current clients include WebMD, *BioWorld Today, BioWorld International, The Lancet Neurology, The Minneapolis Star Tribune,* Newton's Apple, *Current Biology,* BioMedNet, *Annals of Internal Medicine, The Gale Encyclopedias of Science and Mental Health,* The Copley News Service, and The American Chemical Society's Reaction Times He has consulted for American Institutes for Research in Washington, D.C., and Integrated Strategic Information Services, Inc., in California. He is the author of *The Everything Health Guide to Schizophrenia.*

Foreword

There are many books on ophthalmology and eye care that target medical personnel, including practicing ophthalmologists, residents and fellows in ophthalmology, allied ophthalmic personnel, medical students, and non-ophthalmic physicians, among others. Very few publications exist, aside from brochures usually a few pages long published by various entities such as the American Academy of Ophthalmology or produced by physician practices often as promotional material, that address patients and their concerns directly.

Ismail A Shalaby, MD, PhD, and Dean A Haycock, PhD, have now written such a unique, much-awaited, and needed book.

In their book Overcoming Complications of LASIK and Other Eye Surgeries the authors, in a very clear, practical, honest, and unbiased way, discuss various aspects of the eyes and the visual system. The first chapter discusses the anatomy of the eye and explains how its different parts work and interact with the brain in order for us to see. This is a prelude to understanding the chapters that follow. Next are the core chapters of the book in which the authors explain and discuss various ocular conditions and surgeries, including but not limited to refractive surgical procedures, cataracts, glaucoma, and macular degeneration. Readers will learn what to expect before, during, and after many ocular procedures, and the appropriate questions to ask their physicians.

In the last few chapters, the authors tackle very practical, important, and unfortunately often-ignored issues such as how to find and choose the appropriate eye doctor, how to cope with depression caused by vision loss, and low-vision rehabilitation. They also explain the differences between ophthalmologists, optometrists, and opticians. Many physicians would benefit from reading these last few chapters.

The authors conclude with appendices that include a glossary of frequently used terms and various useful resources. Also included in the appendices are examples of some of the consent forms that patients needing treatment will invariably encounter.

Drs. Shalaby and Haycock add a very valuable, practical, and indispensable resource for any individual who either suffers from an eye or visual problem, is considering elective eye surgery (such as LASIK), or just wants to learn more about the way the eyes function and what ailments affect the eyes and how to deal with them.

Ramzi K Hemady, MD
Associate Professor and Acting Chair
Director of Cornea and Uveitis Services
Department of Ophthalmology and Visual Sciences
University of Maryland School of Medicine, Baltimore

Introduction

The authors do not claim or mean to imply that cosmetic corrective eye surgery or other types of ophthalmologic surgeries are generally unsafe. The opposite is true. Overwhelmingly, these procedures are successful: They routinely improve vision and, in many cases, save sight.

Nor do the authors claim that elective eye surgeries should be unquestionably embraced by everyone seeking to rid themselves of glasses or contact lenses. The purpose of this book is to offer information regarding what is and can be done for some of the most common side effects reported after common eye surgeries, including elective procedures.

Writing a book for the general public about this subject may suggest to some readers that these surgeries do more harm than good, a claim made by some outspoken critics of LASIK (laser-assisted *in situ* keratomileusis) and other forms of refractive eye surgery. This is not true. Literally millions of patients are quite happy as a result of their surgeries. For example, a typical patient described his satisfaction with LASIK surgery by noting that it took place five years ago, and, after a year of experiencing mild halos in one eye, his vision is now excellent. "I'm very satisfied," he told us. This patient, like others who share his satisfaction, did not start a Web site to alert readers of the benefits of the procedure that freed him from glasses.

Satisfied medical consumers are generally less likely to seek out people to describe their surgeries to than are discontented ones. People enjoying good outcomes might mention to friends and family that they are impressed and pleased with the results of their operations. Then they generally get on with their lives. For the most part, they don't publicize their results. They don't become advocates for procedures that please them. This is understandable. In the raucous marketplace of public opinion, they are not motivated to be heard above other voices.

In contrast, Web sites abound with complaints from dissatisfied LASIK patients. And it is understandable that patients who are dissatisfied with the results of their operations are motivated to be heard, not silenced. They want relief, their presurgical vision back, and to save other people from experiencing what they experienced. Nothing can negate their legitimate concerns regarding bad outcomes following LASIK or other refractive eye surgery. They have a right to be heard. Indeed, it is important for them to be heard. If you are the person whose eyesight is marred by halos, light sensitivity, or extreme dry eyes to the extent that your life is hampered in a way you could not imagine before your surgery, the fact that most people are happy with their outcomes means little or nothing to you. The complication rate for you is 100 percent.

The fact is, in certain cases, nothing can be done to correct some of the complications following elective eye surgery. In other cases, correction or relief can be obtained with considerable success.

No one knows for certain what the risks or complications are for cosmetic eye surgery procedures such as LASIK. Estimates vary widely. Many doctors who perform the procedure estimate that they are between 1 and 3 percent. The 9,000 or so ophthalmologists represented by The American Society of Cataract and Refractive Surgery (ASCRS), for example, estimate that only 2 to 3 percent of their patients ever experienced complications.

In 2008, the ASCRS claimed, based on close to 3,000 reports published in peer-reviewed medical journal articles, that approximately 95 percent of the 16.4 million people who had LASIK all around the world were happy with their results.

Critics maintain that these figures are the result of surgeons reporting on complications in their own practices, something some doctors might be inclined to underreport. Dissatisfied former patients and activists against these procedures maintain that the complication rate may be 25 percent or higher. This argument might be supported by the report in 2009 that the FDA issued warning letters to 17 LASIK surgical centers that did not, according to the regulatory agency, have an adequate system in place for reporting adverse events. Medical centers that use lasers for LASIK surgery are required to have a written protocol to report when something goes wrong during a procedure.

The problem here is that surgeons are not required to report to the FDA all complaints that *follow* LASIK surgery. The 5-percent-or-less estimate of the incidence of complications might be significantly higher if severe glare, halos, difficulty driving at night, and other issues affecting quality of life after some operations were included in reports of complications that develop during or after surgery. Also, in some cases, 20/20 vision may be the criterion for a successful operation, but difficulty driving at night and other quality-of-life issues may make patients feel they should not be placed in the success column.

Also in 2008, advisors to the FDA may have summarized the true situation concerning controversy surrounding the safety of LASIK surgery when they suggested that the procedure is safe but oversold.[1] The number of contented customers is considerable and far greater than the number of unhappy ones. But in the past, some people who should have been disqualified from having the procedure were instead accepted for treatment. The few irresponsible surgeons who operated on inappropriate patients can not, despite the problems this causes, undo the fact that LASIK surgery appears to be, by and large, a big success and generally a safe procedure for the majority of patients.

The FDA panel chair, Jayne Weiss, MD, of the Kresge Eye Institute in Detroit, said, "The vast majority of patients with LASIK do very well and are very happy and see very well."[1] She agreed that aggressive marketing and treating LASIK as if it were a commodity was a problem. If by commodity she meant the *Merriam-Webster's* definition of "a mass-produced unspecialized product," it would be hard to disagree, if indeed patients who should not have the procedure were encouraged to have it.

Dr. Weiss went on to suggest that problems could be traced to poor patient selection and inadequate informed consent.

An ophthalmologist working for the FDA's Center for Devices and Radiological Health, Malvina Eydelman, MD, told the Raleigh, North Carolina, *News and Observer* that what studies are available "failed to suggest significant problems following LASIK surgery." But, according to the report, Dr. Eydelman also said there was a need for a rigorous study to gather reliable data about complications from this surgery. She told the newspaper, "We also noted that quality-of-life issues related to LASIK had not been evaluated consistently, and there were few reports of well-designed studies."

Despite these concerns, the FDA itself received only 140 comments from people who were dissatisfied with their LASIK surgery during the eight-year period ending in 2006.

The FDA declares on its Web site devoted to LASIK: "Long-term data are not available. LASIK is a relatively new technology. The first laser was approved for LASIK eye surgery in 1998. Therefore, the long-term safety and effectiveness of LASIK surgery is not known."

The FDA, the National Eye Institute, and the United States Department of Defense are collaborating on the LASIK quality-of-life project to determine exactly how voluntary eye surgery impacts the lives of those who have it done. The FDA's interest in this area is related to its responsibility for approving and monitoring the safety of medical devices. In the case of LASIK surgery, that means the different types of laser machines used to reshape patients' corneas.

If successful, the project at last may provide an answer to the question: What percentage of patients suffer debilitating complications as a result of laser surgery? The project will also attempt to document factors present before surgery that can contribute to negative results and dissatisfaction following surgery.

The first phase of the project is designed to gather information from patients using a questionnaire available on the FDA's Web site. Planning began in July 2009. The second phase will also collect information about post-LASIK satisfaction from patients. This part of the project will concentrate on Navy and Marine Corps personnel who receive care at the Navy's Refractive Surgery Center in San Diego, California.

The third and final phase of the project, which might run to 2012 or 2013, will gather information about LASIK satisfaction in individuals across the country in a large, multicenter clinical trial.

The FDA's LASIK Web site is www.fda.gov/MedicalDevices/Products andMedicalProcedures/SurgeryandLifeSupport/LASIK/default.htm.

You can report a problem related to LASIK treatment at www.access data.fda.gov/scripts/medwatch/medwatch-online.htm.

Chapter One

Parts of Your Eye and How They Work

It takes more of your brain's resources to see than it does to hear, smell, feel, or taste. This generous allocation of scarce cerebral real estate reflects the importance of trouble-free eyesight and the dominant role it plays in our lives. Anything that affects our ability to see—nearsightedness, the need for reading glasses, disease, or physical injury—moves to the top of our treatment priority list immediately, with little competition.

Obviously, any surgical procedure that affects the eye is a serious undertaking. This is especially true for a purely cosmetic procedure such as corrective eye surgery. Surgeries that attempt to prevent blindness or restore sight, of course, are just as serious undertakings. But when the consequences of *not undergoing* surgery are worse than the risks of the procedure, it is often easier to accept the possibility, and even the experience, of complications.

In order to understand the potential complications that can occur during and after eye surgery, it is helpful to review the main parts of your eye and how they work together to create the sights you see.

Parts of Your Eye

Each of the main parts of your eye is a highly specialized component of a remarkably sophisticated, yet straightforward, mechanism for seeing. Familiarity with these key structures will help you understand how and why surgical complications happen and how they affect your sight. The eye is shaped roughly like a sphere (see Figure 1.1) with a connecting cable, the optic nerve, linking it to the brain. It is accurate to think of the eye as a direct extension of the brain through which it directly observes its world.

Cornea
The cornea is the clear, dome-shaped part of your eye in front of the colored iris and the lens. It protects the eye and helps focus light coming into it.

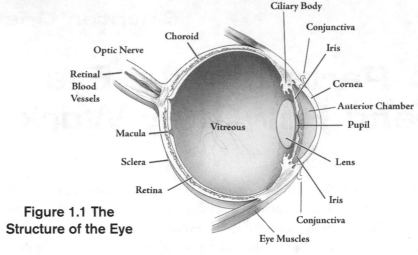

Figure 1.1 The Structure of the Eye

The cornea has no blood supply of its own. If it did, you would look at the world through a tangle of shadowy blood vessels. To spare you this, the cornea depends on diffusion to supply its cells with nutrients and oxygen.

This is one of the reasons the cornea is the most commonly transplanted tissue. It doesn't deteriorate before it is removed from donors and transplanted into recipients' eyes. It is also easily removed for transplantation and available in pairs from donors.

Although the cornea lacks blood vessels, it is rich in pain fibers. This sensitivity allows the eyelid to shut instantly whenever anything like an eyelash or a cinder settles onto the surface of the cornea. Increased tearing stimulated by the presence of a foreign object helps wash it out of the eye.

The cornea appears to be a uniform structure, but it actually consists of several layers. The distinction between these layers is very important for patients of refractive eye surgery. The outermost layer of the cornea is the part that is cut to make a flap of tissue in LASIK surgery. In Photorefractive keratectomy (PRK) surgery, this outermost layer of the cornea is removed.

Just below the outer layer is the middle layer. This is the layer that is shaved or thinned during the LASIK procedure. Finally, there is the deepest corneal layer. This subdivision of the cornea needs to have a certain minimum thickness in order for some surgeries to succeed. If it is too thin, the cornea can fail, become unstable and cloudy, and potentially lead to blindness.

The cornea is a major focusing power in the eye. Along with the natural lens that lies behind it, it allows many fortunate people to see sharply without glasses.

Iris

The cornea covers the iris, the colored part of the eye. The iris acts like a camera shutter to allow light into the back of the eye. In the center of the iris is a hole called the pupil. The size of the pupil is determined by two different sets of muscles that make the opening bigger or smaller. Eye doctors sometimes use chemicals that cause the pupil to become larger. This makes it easier for the doctor to see into the eye.

Trabecular Meshwork

A watery solution, called aqueous humor, is produced in the inner part of the eye and then filtered between the cornea and the iris by internal eye filters. This fluid provides nutrients and oxygen, and removes metabolic waste products for the lens and cornea. It fills the space behind the cornea, the anterior chamber, and the space behind the iris, the posterior chamber.

If this trabecular meshwork of filters is blocked or is slow in draining, pressure builds up in the eye. Prolonged, high eye pressure can cause a condition called glaucoma. Uncontrolled glaucoma can result in loss of peripheral vision, creating tunnel vision and, if untreated, blindness. Its treatments involve methods for reducing the elevated pressure inside the eye.

Under the bone beneath your upper eyelids are the lacrimal glands. They produce tears that keep your eyes moist, wash away dirt, and fight infection. The tears drain out of the eye through tiny holes called puncta. Located in the inside corners of your upper and lower eyelids, puncta drain into the nasal cavity. This explains why crying is also frequently accompanied by a runny nose.

Lens

The lens is a clear, disc-shaped structure. Like the cornea, it contains no blood vessels and gets its nutrients and oxygen through diffusion. Along with the cornea, it plays a key role in focusing light on the retina.

If the lens becomes cloudy, the condition is called a cataract. No longer clear, a lens affected by a cataract does not let enough light into the eye, or it can defocus light that does get in. If a cataract impairs vision to the point of interfering with one's activities, the lens can be removed and replaced with an artificial one.

The focusing ability of the lens is controlled by thin, cable-like ligaments attached to specific muscles. These ciliary muscles contract and pull on the ligaments to change the shape of the lens. Changing the shape of the lens affects how it focuses light. Physicians believe that in your middle-aged years, the lens becomes too stiff to respond to the efforts of this muscle–ligament-focusing mechanism, and you find that you need reading glasses.

Vitreous

Vitreous is a jelly-like material that fills up the back chamber of the eye. It is found behind the lens and is attached to the retina and optic nerve. It often degenerates and separates from the retina, forming clumps that we see as floaters. These are harmless in most cases. Rarely, this separation can tear the retina and lead to a retinal detachment. If you see a sudden large increase in the number of floaters, it might indicate a torn retina. This is an emergency which can often be corrected by prompt surgery.

Unlike the aqueous humor found in the front of the eye, vitreous is not renewed.

Retina

The retina is the sensing part of the eye. It is like the film or light sensor in a camera. Light strikes the retina, which excites retinal cells. These specialized sensory cells send electric signals along nerve fibers through the optic nerve to the brain. The retina contains two main types of sensory cells. Those shaped like cones respond to color and require bright light to work. The others, shaped like rods, work in dim light and respond to movement and shape. They see the world in black, white, and gray.

The center of the retina is called the macula. This is the area where vision is sharpest. Macular degeneration is a condition that results in the destruction of cells in that area, leading to a blur in the center of your vision.

The retina is very handy for physicians. It is literally a window into the circulatory system, providing a way to directly observe blood vessels. It is possible to see the effects of some diseases, including high blood pressure, sickle-cell anemia, high cholesterol, and diabetes, from the damage they produce in blood vessels visible through the retina.

Optic Nerve

The optic nerve is like the electric cable of the eye. It carries electric signals from the 1.5 million or so nerve fibers from the retina to the brain. These nerve fibers are attached to individual, light-sensitive, sensory cells, the rods and cones described above, spread all around the inside of the eyeball in the retina.

Cutting the optic nerve results in complete (dark) blindness. It cannot regenerate or repair itself. Any damage to this bundle of essential nerve fibers, such as that produced by untreated glaucoma, is usually permanent. Prevention and early treatment is essential for any condition or situation that might affect the optic nerve.

In addition to nerve fibers, each optic nerve carries a single artery for delivering blood to the eye and a single vein for returning blood to the lungs where it unloads waste products and picks up fresh nutrients and oxygen. Other organs and structures of the body often have alternative sources of blood supply if one is obstructed. This is not true of the eye (except in very rare cases). Because only one artery delivers blood to the eye, this organ is especially vulnerable to any medical condition that interrupts blood flow in its single artery.

Sclera

If you can see the whites of someone's eyes, you are seeing the sclera. Not transparent like the cornea, the sclera is a hard, protective structure that helps support the globe of the eye by helping to form its outer shell.

One set of cells covers its surface. Unlike the cornea or the lens, this thin layer of clear tissue, called the conjunctiva, contains tiny blood vessels. You can easily see these blood vessels whenever your eyes are bloodshot. If you ever get a red eye, it is usually because the blood vessels of your conjunctiva are inflamed or bleeding. The sclera can sometimes appear blue in people with severe rheumatoid arthritis of the eye because the thinness of the sclera in this condition allows the color of the underlying choroidal layer to show through. The sclera can become inflamed and very painful in rheumatoid arthritis. In rare cases, it can even rupture.

Eye Muscles

Six eye muscles move the eyeball. Two of these muscles move the eyes sideways, two move them straight up or down, and two rotate them. These last two muscles help keep images stationary even when you move your head from side to side. Your nervous system precisely balances the movement of your two eyes, preventing you from seeing two images where there is only one object. Seeing double with both eyes open indicates that the eye muscles or the nerve centers controlling them are out of balance. This might be caused by weak eye muscles, a stroke, a brain aneurysm, multiple sclerosis, or some other medical condition. Sudden double vision with both eyes open should be reported immediately to your doctor, especially if it is accompanied by eye pain or headache. This could imply a brain aneurysm or some other very serious condition.

Visual Brain Cortex

The visual cortex is where all the signals from both eyes are brought together. It is where the brain begins to process and make sense of the visual world. The visual cortex is located far from the eyes, in the rear of the brain, under the back of your skull. It is a long way from the eyes to this essential part of the visual system. This pathway is at risk for strokes, bleeding, swelling, or injury. Neurologists can tell which part of the brain is injured based on what patients experience in their vision. The visual pathways to the brain are crossed, so damage to one side of the brain (such as a stroke), can appear as blindness in the opposite visual field. For example, a stroke in the left part of the visual cortex leads to peripheral-vision blindness in the right half of the visual fields of both eyes.

Basic Optics: How Your Eyes Focus Light to Let You See

Optics is the science of light and how it is focused. Physicists, optometrists, and ophthalmologists have to deal with complex mathematical formulas to gain a solid understanding of optics. Fortunately, you don't need any mathematics to understand the difference between near-, far-, and perfect sight and how refractive surgery or glasses work. However, knowing even a simplified version of visual optics aids in better understanding the complications of LASIK and other surgeries.

Think of light coming from an object you see as straight parallel lines. In order to focus these lines into a clear image, they must be bent so they meet each other at a single point (see figure 1.2). Light rays are bent by a lens. The lens can be a natural lens, your cornea, a lens implant, eye glasses, or contact lenses. The strength needed to bend parallel rays of light to a pinpoint is the power of the lens. If a lens is constructed so that it makes light rays bend farther apart, that is, so the rays separate farther from each other, you will see a blurred image.

Perfect Vision

When the eye is in the shape of a perfect sphere and the focusing power of the cornea and lens are just right, the parallel light rays are focused to a pinpoint on the center of the retina, the area called the macula.

A person lucky enough to have eyes like this does not need glasses for distance viewing. He is said to enjoy perfect sight. Eye doctors call this enviable state of physical health emmetropia.

Nearsightedness

When the eyeball is too long and not perfectly spherical, or when the cornea and/or lens have too much focusing power and bend light too much, nearsightedness or myopia results. In this case, parallel light rays are focused to a point in front of the macula, the target for perfect vision in the center of the retina. Nearsightedness causes faraway objects to look blurry. You have to move closer to them to see them clearly.

This common situation can be corrected by using glasses or contact lenses that bend the light a little farther away from the parallel so they meet at a pinpoint on the macula. With LASIK surgery, the cornea is shaved in such a way that it reduces the focusing power of the cornea by making it bulge less by just the right amount, if everything goes well.

Farsightedness

The opposite of nearsightedness is farsightedness or hyperopia. In this situation, the eyeball is too small, or the cornea and/or lens have too little focusing power. This results in light rays not bending enough. Instead of meeting right where they should for perfect vision on the retina, they meet at a point behind the macula. A person with farsightedness may experience blurred near vision before realizing that her distant vision is blurred as well. Glasses or contact lenses correct this situation by adding more power. LASIK surgery is done in such a way that it adds power to the cornea by making it bulge more.

Astigmatism

Astigmatism occurs if the eyeball is shaped like an American football rather than a sphere. It can also occur if the cornea or the lens is misshapen so that parallel light rays meet not in a single point, but in perpendicular lines. Light rays passing through an astigmatic eye, therefore, do not focus to one point. Astigmatism also often causes

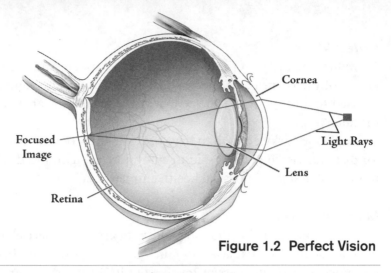

Figure 1.2 Perfect Vision

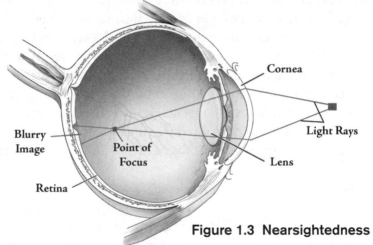

Figure 1.3 Nearsightedness

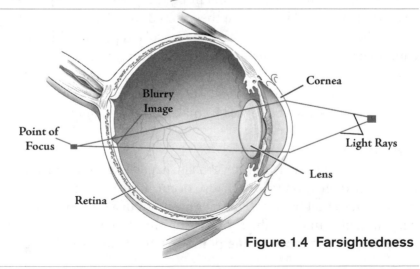

Figure 1.4 Farsightedness

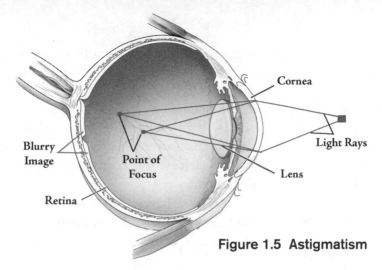

Figure 1.5 Astigmatism

images to appear slanted. Simple astigmatism can be corrected with glasses or contact lenses or through LASIK surgery.

There are conditions called "higher orders of astigmatism," however, in which sparkles and other symptoms appear. These symptoms, unfortunately, are not easy to correct. Sometimes hard (or rigid gas-permeable) contact lenses can minimize the visual distortions by temporarily reshaping the cornea.

Corneal Focusing Power

It comes as a surprise to some people, but the cornea has more focusing power than the lens. This is why the cornea is the center of action in LASIK and PRK refractive eye surgery. If the eye is near-sighted, then LASIK reshapes the cornea to reduce its power by flattening it. If the eye is farsighted, then LASIK reshapes the cornea by making it more pointy or bulgy at its center, therefore increasing its focusing power.

Lens Focusing Power

Think of the first-grade child who wants to show her 45-year-old teacher something she drew. The child shoves the paper 1 inch from the teacher's eyes. The child can see the drawing that close, but the poor teacher has to back up or quickly grab her reading glasses.

Your lenses, at least when you are under the age of 40 or so, can readily adjust their thickness as needed and, therefore, increase or decrease their focusing power. This flexibility enables you to focus easily from far away to up close without glasses. After you reach an age of around 40 years, however, this flexibility decreases enough so that you can no longer easily focus on nearby objects with your unaided eyes. You need reading glasses to compensate for your less flexible lens.

How We See in Three Dimensions

In order for you to have depth perception, or the ability to see in three dimensions, the brain must integrate input from both eyes simultaneously. The visual field of each eye must overlap with the visual field of the other eye in just the right way.

The eyes cannot be crossed or have a significant muscle weakness, and they must have relatively equal vision. If one eye turns in, there will be no depth perception. And, obviously, someone with just one eye has no depth perception.

Of course, you can lack three-dimensional vision without having lost an eye. Having 20/20 vision in one eye and 20/200 vision in the other leaves you with little or no depth perception. This problem can occur when people who need reading glasses choose to use one eye for distance and the other for reading. This is called monovision. Contact-lens wearers often do this. This is also an option for LASIK surgery patients. If the patient cannot tolerate the loss of depth perception after living with the results of her surgery, she may elect to have touch-up LASIK surgery to re-equalize the eyes. If your complications are indeed incapacitating, investigate different types of therapeutic contact lenses described later in this book (Chapter Nine) to determine if any of them might provide relief.

Chapter Two

After Laser Surgery

What's Normal, What's Not and What's Important to Know for Next Time

All corrective eye surgeries are serious procedures and have potential complications. Normal progress toward recovery depends on the type of operation you've had and on your individual response to the changes your eye has experienced. Even with a successful outcome, there is a period of temporary inconvenience. Many of the changes you might experience soon after surgery disappear without treatment as your eye heals in the days, weeks, and months following the procedure.

It is important, however, to understand the difference between normal postoperative changes that occur during this healing/recovery period and complications that might require further medical attention. Knowing the difference between the two allows you to seek early treatment for serious complications, an important step in increasing your chances of getting the best results.

Great (and Unrealistic) Expectations

Some patients feel let down when they realize they have less-than-perfect vision after having elective eye surgery. If you just had LASIK surgery and are anticipating enjoying uncorrected 20/10 vision far and near with both eyes, please adjust your expectations. Chances are you never saw that well with the best pair of glasses or contact lenses you wore at any time before surgery. And you definitely won't see that well after surgery.

The same is true for the person over 40 years of age who used to be moderately nearsighted, never needed bifocals, and merely had to take off his glasses to read the fine print on a medicine bottle. Now, a few weeks after LASIK surgery, he can see the leaves on the trees all the way across the park, but he can no longer make out the writing on an aspirin bottle. Did his doctor let him down? Did she make a mistake during surgery? No, but maybe she didn't discuss, or succeed in getting across to her patient, what he should have expected, and not have expected, following his operation.

No corrective surgery, including LASIK, is or was ever meant to improve visual acuity or the sharpness of vision, beyond what is called "best-corrected" vision. Your best-corrected vision is the best vision your eye can achieve with glasses or soft or rigid gas-permeable contact lenses.

Corrective eye surgery is meant to make you spectacle or contact-lens free, depending on the condition of your eyes before your operation. If your best-corrected vision prior to surgery was 20/10 (and yes, some people can see that well), 20/15, or 20/20, then you should expect successful, uncomplicated, corrective eye surgery to provide the same level of sharpness. If everything goes well, you will achieve it without needing any correction; that is, you'll no longer need glasses or contacts.

If, however, a pre-existing eye condition—a small cataract, a problem with your retina, or a lazy eye, for example—limited your best-corrected vision to, say, 20/40 before corrective surgery, then you should not expect to see better than 20/40 without glasses or contacts following surgery. Your surgeon should explain this *before* operating on you.

Some patients do report better quality of vision after refractive surgery. But if you had certain preoperative vision problems—for example, nearsightedness or farsightedness combined with the inability to focus close-up that usually comes with middle age or the dimness in sight associated with amblyopia—then you may become less dependent on glasses than you were before surgery, but you may still need to wear corrective lenses or contacts.

Consider a person who has a pre-existing eye disease, such as amblyopia or a retinal disease, that prevents her from seeing better than 20/40. In addition, let's say this person is also very near- or farsighted. LASIK treatment may free her from wearing glasses, but she will never see better than 20/40. Or consider a very nearsighted 50-year-old man who wants to reduce the thickness of his glasses, but does not want reading glasses, and would prefer to have nighttime driving glasses. For him, the goal of LASIK surgery would be to under-correct to that appropriate level.

The Qualities of Vision

Often when people think of good eyesight, they think of the familiar concept of 20/20 vision: crisp, clear images and visual acuity. How well you see, however, depends on more than just the sharpness of objects you focus on. It also depends on your ability to see at night and on the presence or absence of irregular astigmatism. It depends on the often underappreciated ability to detect contrasts, handle glare, sense depth, see what is in front of you, and see what is off-center or in your peripheral vision (often called your peripheral visual field).

Ophthalmologists and optical scientists refer to some of the underlying problems affecting these aspects of vision as "higher-order aberrations." It is hard to accurately measure some of these variables, and frankly, they are not well understood. Medical researchers, however, are developing state-of-the-art techniques to help them deal with such problems in the near future.

Treatment, logically, centers on changing or compensating for the specific light-altering irregularities in the eye that cause these visual defects. This can be done by physically altering the cornea with surgery. If surgery is the cause of the aberrations and does not provide further options for correcting them, your options may include custom-made contact lenses orintraocular lens that is surgically implanted to replace the original lens, as is done in cataract surgery.

Beyond Farsightedness, Nearsightedness and Astigmatism

M ost people are familiar with common vision problems, such as farsightedness, nearsightedness, and astigmatism, even if they don't have personal experience with them. The simple diagrams in Chapter One illustrate the basics of these familiar lower-order vision aberrations, which account for approximately 85 percent of overall visual aberrations.

But how many people are as familiar with trefoil, coma, and spherical aberrations, which account for the remaining 15 percent? These higher-order aberrations are unknown to many people and not as easy to picture. Their underlying causes are more complex, and, to make matters even more complicated, people often have more than one of these visual problems at the same time. The lower-order vision deficiencies can be traced to less-than-perfect focusing ability by the cornea and lens. Higher-order deficiencies can be caused by problems with tears, aqueous humor, and vitreous humor, as well as the cornea and lens. Causes include dry eye, irregularly shaped cornea, scarring as a result of injury, disease, surgery, and cataracts.

And they can do more than just make your vision blurry; they can cause you to perceive halos, starbursts, glare, double vision, and to have poor night vision. The effects of these problems can range from mildly distracting or annoying to disabling. People with large pupils may have a greater risk of having higher-order aberration problems than people with average-sized pupils. This is particularly evident in low-light conditions or at night when the pupil expands most. Scarring or other problems that affect the eye's ability to focus light can result in similar problems for people with smaller pupils, too.

Wave-Front Guided LASIK

Custom wave-front guided LASIK is an example of a cutting-edge approach used to correct visual problems that fall in the category of higher-order aberrations, including errors of the eye that produce irregular astigmatism. It also can be used to individualize laser treatment to meet the needs of each eye.

The wave-front guided laser ablation procedure starts with a mathematical description of the shape of your cornea. This sophisticated, complex analysis describes the shape of the cornea with all its variations and irregularities. This data is then programmed into the laser machine to guide it as it corrects many of the irregularities and variations in the corneal surface of each eye. With wave-front guided technology and other advances, higher-order problems of vision may become more amenable to study, manipulation, and correction in the future.

Some surgeons have used wave-front guided lasers for enhancements, or laser re-dos, with good success. Wave-front guidance, however, is not perfect. There have been reports that it still induces higher-order aberrations. Moreover, it tends to remove more tissue than conventional LASIK surgery does. This means people with thin corneas may not be good candidates for this procedure.

The final visual benefits of corrective eye surgery are not immediate. It often can take as long as six months to one year for the eye to recover and stabilize. The speed and quality of recovery depends on the preoperative condition of your eye (the degree and type of your pre-existing visual problem: nearsightedness, farsightedness, astigmatism, presbyopia, dry eye, etc.), the type of refractive surgery you had (PRK, LASIK, and its variations, etc.), the environment in which you live and work (dusty, dry, humid, etc.), and, obviously, the outcome of the surgery (uncomplicated versus complicated).

Informed Consent

Refractive eye surgery is cosmetic surgery: It is not medically necessary. Before the procedure, you had a normal eye that required glasses or contact lenses, and you asked an eye surgeon to perform an invasive procedure on it. As with any type of surgery, refractive eye surgery comes with risks. Typically, these risks are small but very real. You, and not your surgeon, have to weigh the risks—as explained to you by the surgeon or your eye doctor—against the benefits. Then you come up with a decision. This process is called "informed consent," because you should have been informed and, after careful consideration, you consented or agreed to the procedure with all its associated risks.

A good informed-consent interaction between you and your eye surgeon involves a face-to-face discussion regarding the risks, benefits, and alternatives to the procedure, the typical postoperative course, and the expected outcome. If you decide to have surgery, take the informed-consent document or pamphlet home, read it carefully, and make sure all of your questions are answered to the best of the surgeon's abilities. Then sign it and return it to your doctor's office before your surgery.

An example of a poor informed-consent interaction would be if your surgeon or his assistant handed you a piece of paper listing everything that could happen during and after the procedure and then asked you to sign it 30 minutes before surgery. To an ethical ophthalmologist, an informed consent document is not a piece of paper designed to legally protect him from being sued (which it may fail to do anyway). It is a way for your doctor to know that you fully understand what will happen and what can go wrong during and after the procedure.

The best time to ask questions about potential complications is during the discussion of the information in the informed-consent material. Be wary of a surgeon who tells you that she has never had any complications. That surgeon is either lying or has not yet performed enough surgeries to have experienced complications in her patients.

Because doctors are human, they do, sometimes, have patients with complications. Some complications are caused by lack of experience or skill; many other complications are the result of statistical chance. One necessary skill of a good surgeon is to know how to get a good outcome from a bad complication. We have included in the appendix an example of a good informed-consent form. No matter what informed-consent document you receive, it should not be a substitute for an informed discussion.

After Eye Surgery

Obviously, it is normal to feel some discomfort and less-than-perfect vision immediately after undergoing eye surgery. In most cases, these problems get better if you follow the procedures for caring for your eyes provided to you by your ophthalmologist.

Right after surgery, your eyes may water, burn, or itch, and your vision may be blurred. Other, expected consequences of surgery may last for days, weeks, or even months. If any of the following normal, postoperative developments fail to resolve themselves and last longer than your doctor predicted, make an appointment with that doctor. If the following problems continue to bother you after further consultation with your original doctor, get another opinion:
  • moderate or mild blurred vision
  • scratchy eye
  • dry eye
  • night-vision problem
  • glare
  • halos

Serious Complications

In a minority of cases, serious symptoms that fall outside the category of normal, expected sensations and problems develop or linger too long after surgery. They are clear indications that something requires immediate medical intervention. They may be the result of infection, a bad reaction to medication, or unanticipated and unfortunate damage to the cornea or other part of the eye. Do not hesitate to contact your doctor if you experience the following symptoms.

These postsurgical symptoms should send you back to your doctor *immediately*:
- severe unrelenting eye pain
- extreme light sensitivity
- sudden blurred vision
- double vision
- eye discharge accompanying infection
- nausea/vomiting

The following are some other complaints that also require a trip to the ophthalmologist for surgical touch-up, prescription lenses, or other adjustments *after your eye has healed completely*:
- nearsightedness, if you were farsighted before surgery
- farsightedness, if you were nearsighted before surgery
- progressive blurred vision after your apparently successful surgery (regression)

To determine whether your experience after surgery is normal or not, we review the potential pitfalls that can accompany common refractive surgery procedures. This information should have been explained to you by your doctor or spelled out clearly in the informed consent guide that you signed before surgery. Refamiliarizing yourself with its main points may reassure you about the course of the healing process you are experiencing or, depending on your symptoms, help you avoid unhappy surprises following future and touch-up surgery, if that is what you decide to have.

As discussed, your expectations of the refractive surgery should be realistic. If you wore glasses and have some sort of eye disease that limits your vision to less than 20/20 at a distance—and assuming that pre-existing vision problem did not pose a high risk with the refractive surgery—you can expect to see without glasses or contacts just as well as you saw with them, but no better. The laser surgery was intended to free you of your need for corrective lenses, not to cure your eye disease.

Recovery and Your Options for Treating Complications after Refractive Eye Surgeries

Common elective procedures to correct poor vision are variations of a single strategy: They reshape the surface of the cornea to change the way it focuses images on the retina. The curvature of the cornea is adjusted using a concentrated beam of light or an ultraviolet laser. The energy of this particular type of ultraviolet light is limited and poses no threat to any part of the eye except the surface of the cornea that is being reshaped. The techniques differ mostly in the way a surgeon gains access to the surface of the cornea that needs to be reshaped to improve vision.

What Are the Differences Between Types of Refractive Surgery?

Before a laser can reshape the cornea to improve its focusing ability, a thin layer of epithelial cells that lie on the surface of the cornea must be removed or moved aside. Different laser surgery procedures with unfortunately similar and confusing names use different methods of exposing the cornea.

PRK involves scraping the epithelial cell layer off the corneal surface. The epithelial cells regrow by themselves within a week, but the epithelial cell layer itself takes longer to recover.

Epi-LASEK involves the use of alcohol to soften and lift the epithelium off the cornea. The epithelium can be replaced after the laser work is done. The alcohol, however, takes a little toll on the viability of the epithelial cells, but they can recover nicely.

Epi-LASIK uses a very sharp, precise cutting instrument to slice a thin layer of the epithelium to create a flap that is moved aside and replaced.

LASEK uses a blade to create a flap of epithelial tissue and then alcohol to loosen it and lift it out of the way.

LASIK also uses a blade to create a flap, but it involves a deeper cut that lifts the epithelium and reaches into the middle layer of the cornea as well.

PRK

The first technique developed to correct poor vision by reshaping (doctors call it ablating) the surface of the cornea with laser energy was PRK (photorefractive keratectomy). It involves physically scraping off the thin, outermost layer of cells on the surface of the cornea, the epithelium, to expose the underlying layer called the stroma. Unlike other laser procedures, PRK does not involve the creation of a thin flap of corneal tissue, which is moved aside to allow access to the deeper cornea before being replaced.

Because the epithelium is removed and not replaced, it can take weeks or even months for vision to recover completely following PRK. A bandage contact lens protects the eye while the epithelial layer regrows (usually in a week).

PRK can be more uncomfortable than some other procedures, and healing times may vary.

While it is not as popular, or performed as often, as LASIK surgery, PRK has distinct advantages over LASIK for some people. For example, it is not as dependent on corneal thickness as the LASIK procedure is, because it does not involve the creation of a flap. Therefore, patients with thin corneas who are ineligible for LASIK may be eligible for PRK. In addition, unlike the LASIK procedure, the PRK procedure does not include a step that uses suction, which creates a brief period of high eye pressure. This means people who have mild glaucoma or high eye pressure may still be eligible for PRK refractive eye surgery when LASIK is not an option for them.

The exact healing time depends on the individual and how much correction was required. It takes longer to heal if you were very near-sighted. The more corneal tissue removed during the laser procedure, the greater the risk of scarring. This can result in surface haze, an annoying problem that usually goes away on its own in six months or so. Corneal haze typically peaks a couple of months after PRK and then gradually resolves itself. To lessen this complication in at-risk patients, PRK surgeons add an antimetabolite chemical called mitomycin C during the procedure. Mitomycin C inhibits cell division and scar formation. Since corneal haze is a result of scarring, mitomycin C is helpful in this situation. If corneal haze does occur after PRK, retreatment with PRK (then called PTK [phototherapeutic keratectomy] because it is therapeutic, not cosmetic), and mitomycin C may also be effective.

Sometimes, patients may notice changes in their ability to focus. This problem also often eases and vision stabilizes by itself. Your doctor may prescribe steroids if you show signs of this problem.

Watch for signs of infection and inflammation in the weeks and months following your PRK surgery. These are usually easily treated with antibiotics or steroids.

Finally, PRK can be re-done if the outcome isn't satisfactory the first time.

Epi-LASEK

Epi-LASEK (laser epithelial keratomileusis) is a version of PRK which has the same complications and risks. Epi-LASEK differs from PRK only in the way the epithelium on the surface of the cornea is removed before the laser is brought in to reshape the surface of the cornea. It is a hybrid procedure in which the epithelium is briefly soaked in dilute alcohol before a flap is created with an instrument called an epikeratome. Instead of being scraped off as it is in PRK, the layer of epithelial cells included in the flap is lifted off in Epi-LASEK. This procedure was developed with the intention of decreasing the postoperative pain associated with PRK as well as the chances of developing corneal haze.

The exposed cornea is reshaped with the laser, and the epithelium is then gently placed into its original position. If for some reason the alcohol-treated epithelium does not survive the procedure, it can be discarded. When this happens, the Epi-LASEK procedure essentially becomes a PRK procedure.

If the epithelium is not pretreated with alcohol, the procedure is called Epi-LASIK.

Epi-LASIK

In the Epi-LASIK (epithelial laser *in situ* keratomileusis) procedure, the epithelium is moved aside, not by scraping, but by precision cutting. The surgeon uses a precise cutting instrument, called a microtome, to create a very thin slice of the epithelium that is then folded back. This differs from the LASIK flap-cutting procedure described in the next section because it does not involve cutting any of the middle portions of the cornea lying just beneath the outermost epithelial layer. The idea is that by avoiding use of alcohol, which can irritate epithelial cells a little, and by not cutting into the stromal layer of the cornea, less damage will be done to the eye as the cornea is being prepared for laser treatment.

Epi-LASIK has been more successful, and is now used more frequently, than LASEK. So far, however, follow-up studies have not shown that LASEK or Epi-LASIK have lower risks of corneal haze complications than PRK.

LASEK

LASEK (laser epithelial keratomileusis) involves the creation of a hinged flap of tissue covering the cornea. LASEK was developed in an attempt to reduce the postsurgical pain associated with PRK and its associated complication rate of corneal haze. The surgeon uses a blade called a trephine to create a flap of epithelial tissue. In this procedure, however, the flap of tissue is treated with alcohol, which lifts it up and away from the surface of the eye. As always, the surgeon gently sets the flap aside to open the way for the laser to reshape the corneal surface. LASEK does not involve an incision into the cornea as LASIK surgery does.

Although technically more demanding, this procedure has not been shown to offer substantial improvement over PRK. Several studies suggest that vision on the first postoperative day may be better, but this initial improvement may not last. There have been complications with flap loss, or sloughing off of the epithelial layer, due to the thinness of the flap.

It may take longer to recover from LASEK surgery than it does from LASIK surgery. It also may be a bit more painful, but there are fewer complications related to the creation of the corneal flap because it has no corneal flap to begin with; only epithelial tissue is included in the flap created during this procedure. Blurry vision, dry eyes, poor low light and night vision, and other visual aberrations are usually short-lived and should be gone after six months or a year. If they linger longer than that, discuss the options described on pages 39 and 42 with your doctor.

LASIK

LASIK (laser-assisted *in situ* keratomileusis) differs from PRK and Epi-LASEK in the way the epithelium is treated before the laser reshapes the cornea. It does not rely on scraping the epithelial cells off as PRK does. It does not involve the use of alcohol to loosen them as Epi-LASEK does. Instead, it relies on the use of a precise cutting tool, called a microkeratome, to create a hinged flap consisting of epithelium and a thin portion of the underlying corneal tissue, called stromal tissue.

An important difference between LASIK and PRK is the use of suction to stiffen the cornea temporarily to ease precise flap formation. This suction by necessity temporarily raises the eye pressure to very high levels. This has the potential of harming patients who already have high eye pressure.

It is also possible to create a thin flap of epithelial/corneal tissue using a laser controlled by a computer instead of using a microkeratome. This is called femtosecond laser or Intralase.

This specialized laser can cut through the cornea to create a flap in a very precise way. Many eye surgeons believe this may avoid some of the potential complications of the microtome, such as free-flaps and uneven cutting, which are discussed later in this chapter.

The flap created by the blade or laser is moved aside and replaced after the cornea is reshaped. A protective eye shield, antibiotics, and anti-inflammatory medications protect the eye during the immediate postrecovery phase.

You may notice better vision as quickly as one or two weeks after surgery with LASIK. For some people, vision may not stabilize completely for as long as six months, but recovery time is generally shorter than it is with PRK. Because the flap of tissue created during LASIK includes epithelial tissue and some corneal tissue, however, the cornea may actually be a little weaker for years after surgery, until healing is 100-percent complete.

Medical Reasons *Not* to Have LASIK Surgery

Any medical reason that you should not have a particular type of surgery or treatment is called a contraindication. Physicians classify your risks of developing complications into two categories: relative and absolute contraindications. A relative contraindication means you are at risk for developing a complication but are likely to do well if you and your doctor anticipate it and take steps to prevent it. An absolute contraindication is one that should prevent you from having surgery even if you and your doctor can anticipate the likely complication.

The combination of extreme nearsightedness and a much thinner-than-normal cornea is an absolute contraindication for LASIK: You are not eligible for LASIK if you have these conditions.

After LASIK surgery, the center of your cornea must be at least 250 microns thick. (One micron equals 0.001 millimeters.) If it is thinner than that, you could end up needing a corneal transplant.

If one LASIK surgeon hesitates to perform LASIK surgery on you and a second assures you it is safe, trust the first, and seek a third opinion. Don't let your desire to see without glasses lead you to make a bad decision. Find out if you are eligible for clear lens extraction, an alternative procedure that is not dependent on corneal thickness. You will still have to balance the advantages and disadvantages of this alternative, of course; extreme nearsightedness, for example, increases the risk of developing a retinal detachment following clear lens extraction.

If you are nearsighted and have a high degree of astigmatism, you may have keratoconus—a thin, bulging cornea—or a related corneal disorder. This is another absolute contraindication; if your ophthalmologist says you have keratoconus, you should not undergo LASIK. Keratoconus can be diagnosed clinically, but it can also be easily picked up by corneal topography, one of the basic measurements performed prior to refractive surgery. To the ophthalmologist, the presence of keratoconus is a *stop* sign for LASIK or PRK. This condition is obvious to your surgeon when he examines your cornea, and he'll tell you that you cannot have LASIK. You may, however, be eligible for intrastromal ring segments, such as Intacs (discussed in Chapter Nine).

If you have had corneal transplant surgery, you may have astigmatism and be nearsighted as well. Be careful if you are considering LASIK surgery. Results following LASIK among people who have had corneal transplants are not as successful as they are among people who have not had a transplant. Although the transplant itself may become unstable after LASIK, a history of corneal transplantation, nevertheless, is not an absolute contraindication for LASIK. Discuss this carefully with your ophthalmologist.

A history of cold sores in the cornea (herpes infection) or shingles is a relative contraindication for LASIK. If you haven't had a recurrence of the infection for years, then you will probably be okay, with only a minimal risk of reactivation of these viruses. If, on the other hand, you have had recurrences, make sure your surgeon knows the details. This may make you ineligible for this type of surgery, because the laser light that is used or the actual trauma of the flap formation theoretically may reactivate the virus. Also, a past herpes or zoster virus corneal infection may leave your corneal nerves less sensitive to pain and irritation. This impaired nerve function may, in turn, increase your risk of developing a dry eye. Additionally, the steroid drops that are given after LASIK may also increase the risk of reactivating the latent viruses. Fortunately, patients who experience a reactivation of these infections following LASIK have been successfully treated with antiviral eyedrops or pills.

If you have had a history of high eye-pressure or are being treated for glaucoma, losing peripheral vision or worsening the glaucoma is a risk. Part of the LASIK procedure involves keeping your eye steady as the flap is created. This is done using suction, which brings the eye pressure up to 65 mm Hg—a very high reading. If your optic nerve is healthy, it will not suffer damage with this pressure as long as it lasts only a few minutes. If, however, your optic nerve is damaged by glaucoma, the high-pressure–inducing suction associated with LASIK may further damage the nerve. Optic-nerve damage from such high eye-pressure is not reversible; you could lose peripheral vision, and nothing can be done about that. It is best to be safe and not have LASIK if you have a history of high eye-pressure or are being treated for glaucoma. Up to a quarter of nearsighted people have glaucoma, so you must be careful if you are considering LASIK. As always, if you are not satisfied, get a second opinion.

Ask if you are eligible for PRK if you can't have LASIK, because PRK does not involve suction that produces high eye pressure. However, steroid drops, which can greatly increase eye pressure, are routinely used after both PRK and LASIK, so discuss this with your surgeon as well.

Some Reasons Not to Have LASIK Surgery

Discuss with your ophthalmologist your eligibility for refractive eye surgery, and consider alternative solutions and options to improve your eyesight if:
- you are extremely nearsighted
- you have a thin cornea
- you have a particularly wide pupil
- your cornea is abnormally shaped
- you have a disease that affects your immune system or you are taking immunosuppressive drugs
- you have diabetes
- you have glaucoma or have had a corneal transplant
- you have had serious eye infections
- you have had retinal tears or detachments
- you have persistent dry eyes

You should get a retinal surgeon's opinion before having LASIK or refractive eye surgery if you have experienced a retinal tear or detachment in the past. It might increase your risk of having another tear or detachment as can clear lens extraction. A retinal specialist may treat any low-risk retinal tears with "spot-weld" lasers as a precaution before your refractive surgery. If you are thinking of getting a multifocal premium lens implant, be sure your retinal specialist examines you very carefully beforehand. Subtle retinal changes (such as epiretinal membranes, discussed in Chapter Twelve) that may not be obvious to a LASIK surgeon can become very visually annoying to someone who has had multifocal premium lens implants—so annoying that these lenses often have to be removed and exchanged with standard monofocal lens implants.

If you have amblyopia, or lazy eye, make sure your expectations from LASIK are realistic. While the procedure may succeed in reducing the thickness of your glasses, your affected eye will not have perfect 20/20 or 20/10 vision.

Some farsighted people's eyes turn inward, a condition known as strabismus. When they get prescription glasses, their strabismus is corrected. If these same people get LASIK surgery to correct their farsightedness, their eyes may once again turn inward. If you have this problem, your doctor should examine your eye muscles and their strength carefully before you undergo LASIK.

Other health conditions, some common and some not, must be taken into consideration if you are thinking about LASIK. Diabetes, for instance, hinders your ability to heal. In one study, almost half of the patients with diabetes who received PRK or LASIK surgery had a high incidence of complications. If you are HIV positive, the addition of steroid drops after LASIK could make it even more difficult for your immune system to fight infection. Not many studies have been done in this area, but you should definitely consult your infectious disease doctor and your family doctor before LASIK surgery.

Another disease, rheumatoid arthritis, and related arthritis-like inflammatory diseases, pose a different type of risk. Autoimmune diseases such as these may put you at risk of corneal melt, a degeneration of your cornea following LASIK. Do not have LASIK if you are suffering from one of these diseases. Do not have the surgery if you are taking medications that suppress your immune system. If, however, your rheumatoid arthritis is well-controlled, your risk of developing complications is not higher than it is for other people undergoing the operation. You also have the option of considering clear-lens extraction instead of LASIK.

It is possible to have sharp vision after LASIK surgery—20/20 or even 20/15—and still have complications such as dry eyes and sensitivity to light, glare, and halos. Additional surgery or medication may help correct or relieve these problems (see Sidebar). Other complications include irregular astigmatism and unclear vision.

If the surgery over- or under-corrected your vision problem, you might be able to correct the less-than-perfect result by wearing glasses when needed. If the over- or under-correction is considerable, you may benefit from a repeat surgery. The surgeon should be able to lift the flap made during the first surgery to re-do the job. Infections are rare, and if they do occur, they are treated with antibiotics.

Potential LASIK Eye Surgery Problems and Treatments

- Night-vision problems taking the form of starbursts, double vision, glare, and/or halos. These might improve with short-term use of corticosteroid eyedrops. If that doesn't solve the problem, more surgery sometimes does.

- Dry eyes may annoy you for up to six months following surgery, during which time you can use eyedrops recommended by your doctor. If the problem is severe and persists, you can consider having plugs put into the tear-draining ducts in your eye to increase tear levels. In serious cases of dry eye, you may have to use artificial tears long-term.
- Astigmatism, a type of blurry vision caused by a less-than-smooth corneal surface where tissue has been removed, might be corrected with another operation.
- Improper healing of the flap created during laser surgery also may require additional surgery.
- Under-correction results when not enough corneal tissue has been removed. After your eyes have healed, this may be fixed with a second operation.
- Overcorrection results from the removal of too much corneal tissue. More difficult to fix with touch-up surgery, this condition may require glasses or contact lenses.

Induced astigmatism is another rare complication of LASIK surgery. It is the result of scarring that leaves the cornea warped enough to distort or blur images. Contact lenses won't help correct this problem, but glasses often can provide better vision.

Flap Problems

A greater source of complications, when they occur, can be traced to problems with the flap created to expose the cornea. When replaced, the flap may develop wrinkles or folds. Fortunately, these usually are not difficult for your eye surgeon to see and smooth out.

Sometimes, the laser treatment leaves bumps on the treated surface of the cornea. The visual distortions caused by these bits of uneven tissue, called central corneal islands, may correct themselves in a month or two. If they persist, one option to explore is prescription contact lenses. For others, additional surgery can smooth out the irregularities.

Surgical adjustment may also be required if your vision after LASIK is impaired by epithelial cells growing where they aren't supposed to be growing: under the corneal flap.

These epithelial ingrowths may stop growing on their own, but if they don't, additional surgery, in which the flap is raised and the wayward cells are removed, can take care of this complication.

After surgery, it is possible for the cornea under the flap to become inflamed beyond what you would expect as a result of the surgery itself. There are many causes. If small particles or foreign bodies found their way under the flap, for example, this serious condition, called diffuse lamellar keratitis (DLK), could occur. It usually happens in a matter of days after surgery. However, if you suffer an eye injury, even years after surgery, you can still get DLK. Your vision may be blurred. You may be sensitive to light, feel pain, and feel as if you have something in your eye. Anytime you injure your eye—even if you think you are okay—have it checked by an eye care professional.

Your eye doctor can spot this problem during checkups, even if you don't have any of the typical symptoms after your surgery. DLK can often be treated effectively with medication—antibiotics and steroids—if detected soon enough. In some cases, it may be necessary to lift the flap and clean the underlying cornea to correct the problem.

Another serious complication results in a bulging cornea. If the flap created during the operation included too much corneal tissue, or if the laser removed too much of the cornea, the cornea can be weakened. This complication is called keractisia. The misshaped cornea distorts the image, since it can no longer focus effectively on your retina. Your options may include using gas-permeable contact lenses or special corneal implants called Intacs to hold the bulging cornea in place.

A novel approach to treating this condition involves the use of eyedrops containing vitamin B_2, which is also known as riboflavin. Exposed to ultraviolet light, the riboflavin in the eyedrops interacts with the connective tissue fibers that make up the cornea. This chemical interaction makes the points of contact between the connective tissue fibers stronger. If it works, the structure of the cornea is enhanced, the corneal weakness lessened, and the bulging stopped. This technique is known as C3-R. The Cs stand for corneal collagen cross-linking, and the R for riboflavin.

If C3-R does a good job of strengthening the cornea, it may even be possible to perform touch-up surgery, something that would be out of the question with untreated cases of keractisia.

Finally, you may have the option of a corneal transplant if your thin cornea is too unstable.

Dry Eyes

Another potential problem is well-known but still sometimes overlooked before laser surgery: the dry eye. Many patients who seek consultation for refractive surgery can no longer comfortably wear, or have become tired of wearing, contact lenses. Typically they cannot wear their lenses for extended periods of time, or they frequently have to apply lubricants or rewetting drops to keep their eyes comfortable. These are typical signs of someone with a tear-film deficiency or dry eyes.

This condition greatly increases the risk of experiencing problems following vision-correction surgery. These patients often have to be treated for dry eyes prior to the surgery. They may need to use artificial teardrops or medicated eyedrops for the rest of their lives. Another option for some of them is the use of punctal plugs, which are very tiny "corks" that block the pores through which tears normally drain from the surface of the eye. The plugged exit routes allow the tears that are produced to remain in the eye longer and help lubricate its surface.

Dry eye may also become a problem for you after surgery even if your eyes were well lubricated before surgery. If you experience dry eye after LASIK surgery, your doctor may suggest you use artificial tears, or she may prescribe a medication to treat the problem. Taking flaxseed and omega-3 fish oil capsules may also help. If your eyes are still dry after six months or longer, blocking the drainage of tears from the eye with punctal plugs may be an option worth considering. Dry eyes are discussed in more detail in Chapter Three.

Potential Remedies to Discuss with Your Doctor

There are no guarantees that the remedies available for treating complications of eye surgery will help you, but you should discuss all of the possibilities with your doctor. If you experience ghosting or double vision, see halos or starbursts, experience glare, poor vision in low light, including nighttime, or have decreased ability to see contrasts, there may be steps you can take which might relieve your symptoms. The success of these approaches, of course, depends on the exact nature of your vision problem and the condition of your eye and general health. Some potential remedies to consider are:

- Glasses or contact lenses may help if you have blurry vision or don't see well, your surgery under- or overcorrected your vision, you have residual astigmatism, or the improvement you enjoyed after your surgery fades and your vision reverts to what it was before you had surgery.

- Surgical touch-up or laser retreatment may help correct some of the visual aberrations listed above as well as haze. It also can correct some irregularities left on the laser-treated cornea that produce these irritating problems.

- Surgical flap adjustment/cleaning involves lifting, smoothing out, and replacing the flap, and it can often correct problems caused by a less-than-smooth flap surface, including folds and wrinkles.

- Surgical flap rinsing/cleaning involves lifting the flap and physically removing material, including epithelial cells, that shouldn't be present on the surface of the cornea. This effective cleaning procedure also may be useful in treating inflammation in some cases.

- Eyedrops prescribed by your doctor may help you deal with many complications, including dry eyes, some visual aberrations caused by oversized pupils, inflammation (DLK), and infection.

- Oral antibiotics may be used to treat infections and tear imbalance.

- Oral flaxseed and omega-3 fish oils may relieve the irritation, itching, and redness associated with dry eye.

- Punctal plugs can be inserted by a doctor into your eyes' tear-duct drainage holes to increase the amount of tears on the surface of your eye and help counter dry eye.

Sometimes It's about Tradeoffs

Remember the 40-something man described earlier who found he could no longer see fine print after surgery as well as he could before? He had been moderately nearsighted prior to his procedure. This protected him from the initial stage of that middle-aged rite of passage, presbyopia, which makes reading glasses necessary. His successful LASIK surgery corrected his need for distance glasses and eliminated his nearsightedness, the very thing that allowed him to read fine print while his middle-aged friends were reaching for their reading glasses. After successful surgery, he is no longer slightly nearsighted, he has lost his protection from presbyopia and now needs reading glasses. If he hadn't been informed of this fact in advance, he may have been disappointed to learn that he has traded his distance glasses for reading glasses.

Another trade-off to keep in mind is that eye surgery often improves or saves your vision but rarely results in perfect vision. This is because no one has perfect eyes, either before or after surgery. Some lucky people have great vision, and some patients have excellent vision after surgery, but visual aberrations are probably not as rare as many people think. People have varying degrees of higher-order visual aberrations. Some people may have more aberrations after surgery than they had before. But the degree of their postsurgical visual aberrations might equal those of someone who can live quite happily with the same degree of visual impairment because that person has always lived with it. Though moderate starbursts and halos, for example, are not debilitating, they may weigh much more on someone who is not used to them than they do on someone who has learned to live with them.

No one would argue that you have a serious postsurgical complication if you have lost the ability to drive at night following laser eye surgery. But if you have less serious complications, such as seeing starbursts and halos that don't prevent you from driving, you might learn to ignore them as many people do. Expecting perfect vision, when few people have that ability, can lead to unnecessary frustration.

Chapter Three

More About LASIK and Its Complications
Dry Eyes and Other Tearing Problems

If you spoke Greek, you would recognize the phrase "cornea carving" in LASIK's full name: laser *in situ* keratomileusis, since kerato means cornea, and mileusis means carving. Today, this method of cornea carving is by far the most popular of the refractive eye surgeries. It is, in the opinion of many doctors and patients, the safest, most effective, and most comfortable procedure with the shortest recovery time.

During LASIK surgery, a specialized, very sharp-cutting blade called a microtome is used to create a hinged flap out of a portion of the cornea. The flap includes the outer layer of epithelial cells and the more superficial part of the middle stromal layer of the cornea. With the flap lifted and set aside, the stromal layer of the cornea is treated with the laser until the proper, predetermined shape and thickness is attained. The hinged flap is then put back into its original place. Natural forces, produced by osmotic pressure and other features of the cornea, help the flap stay in place after it has been repositioned.

Surgical complications that can occur with LASIK or Intralase (the version of LASIK that uses a laser instead of a blade to create the flap) typically involve the formation of the corneal flap. If the surgeon notices a "free flap," one that is missing a hinge and is therefore free to move, surgery is continued and the flap is sewn in place. A bandage contact lens is placed temporarily on the eye.

If the flap is uneven and thin, or if it has a hole in it (a condition called "button holing"), the flap is, again, put back in place. Then the cornea is allowed to heal for several months. The patient wears a bandage contact lens for a week or so. After the eye has healed, it may be possible to try surgery once again.

Blurred vision may result if wrinkles form on the underside of the flap. This happens occasionally. The wrinkles are situated over the part of the cornea that has been thinned by the laser. Various factors can lead to wrinkling, but, as with misalignment, early recognition of the problem makes it relatively easy to correct this complication. Your surgeon can reposition the flap and smooth out the wrinkles.

Other more serious complications include a lost flap, something that could happen with older microtomes. If the corneal flap was caught in these now-obsolete instruments, the tissue could be destroyed.

Corneal perforation—an extremely rare event—could be devastating. A corneal perforation can result if too much material is removed and the laser penetrates beyond the middle layer of the cornea into its deeper layers. It is important to stress that this is a highly unlikely complication and is one associated with instruments no longer in use.

What to Expect the First Week after LASIK Surgery

At this point in your recovery, your uncorrected vision should be much better than it was before the surgery, but not at its final, stable point yet. You are using antibiotic and steroid eyedrops with the addition of frequent lubricating drops, which serve as artificial tears. This may continue for a week or more, depending on the extent of your surgery and on the dryness of your eyes.

On your first postoperative day, your surgeon checks the corneal flap and makes sure it is stable and in proper position. She also checks for any signs of infection and abnormal inflammation. Also, you will probably be asked to wear goggles while showering and sleeping to protect the corneal flaps from accidental movement.

Complications that can occur during this period, again, most often affect the flap. It can become decentered, misaligned, or sloughed off. For these reasons, do not rub or touch your eyes. Misalignment of the flap is not rare, and its main symptom is blurred vision. If you or your doctor recognizes it in the first few days, the flap can be repositioned relatively easily by the surgeon.

The epithelial layer of the cornea can be eroded, or the cornea can be scraped or abraded, if the microtome rubs against its surface. Typical symptoms are eye pain and increased sensitivity to light. These complications would be recognized on your first postoperative visit and would be treated with a bandage contact lens and artificial tears. People over age 35 are more prone to these problems. Also, people with dry eyes (see below) or certain epithelial cornea problems are at higher risk for epithelial erosions. If not treated, these can often lead to recurrent epithelial erosions.

As with any surgical procedure, infection is a potential complication. In the case of LASIK surgery, fortunately, it is a rare complication. The symptoms are pain, discharge, and blurred vision. Infections can occur as soon as two to three days, or as late as two weeks, after surgery. Usually bacteria are associated with early infections and fungi and yeast with later infections. Both need to be treated aggressively; otherwise the cornea can be destroyed.

An inflammatory condition caused by chemicals and possible contaminants can occur as soon as one day after surgery. This condition, DLK, may require flap irrigation and repositioning. Another potential problem is epithelial ingrowth in which epithelial cells from the corneal surface layer slip under the flap and begin growing deep in the cornea where they don't belong. This very serious complication needs to be treated aggressively or it can blur vision permanently by clouding the normally clear cornea.

What to Expect Beyond the First Two Weeks after LASIK Surgery

After three to six months, if everything goes well, your vision should have improved to its final, expected level. This is a shorter interval than seen with PRK surgery, in which the epithelial layer is scraped away and must grow back. If your surgery was a complete success, you should no longer need glasses for distance vision. Your eyesight should be equally good in the day and night with no glare or halos (unless, as previously explained, you had those symptoms before surgery).

Unless you have dry eyes, lubricating drops should be discontinued three months after surgery. Steroid drops, depending on the extent of your laser treatment, also may have been discontinued by this time. All your normal activities should have resumed with no restriction on swimming or the use of hot tubs (these are restricted during the first two to four weeks following surgery). If, after three months, you still need some distance correction to see your best, this would be the time to consider enhancement or touch-up surgery.

Ghosting of images and double or triple vision indicate you might have central islands or bumps in the part of the cornea that has been laser-treated. Another complication that can show up after two weeks is epithelial ingrowth. Halos and glare at night can be traced to a wide pupil, the edges of which extend past the outer edges of the adjusted cornea, the laser ablation zone. Irregular astigmatism and other problems grouped under the category of higher-order visual errors can also become apparent this late after surgery.

PRK, the oldest of these surgical procedures, has lower risks of causing glare and halos than LASIK does, but both procedures may increase irregular astigmatism.

Long-term use of steroid drops can increase eye pressure and cause glaucoma with possible loss of peripheral vision. This can be missed because the thin cornea resulting from LASIK or PRK gives a falsely low eye-pressure measurement when traditional methods of eye-pressure testing are used. This means high eye pressure, the cause of glaucoma, may escape notice.

Corneal transplants may be necessary in the extremely rare event that corneal swelling and clouding occurs. Other very rare complications include retinal bleeding and optic nerve strokes following laser refractive surgery. The mechanisms behind many of these highly unlikely complications are not understood.

Dry Eyes

Catchall phrases, including dry eye, dry eyes, dry eye syndrome, dysfunctional tear syndrome, and keratoconjunctivitis sicca, are all used to describe different tear and eyelid problems. Symptoms may include red, burning eyes, a gritty feeling on the cornea, the sensation that something is in your eye, and, ironically, tearing and the production of thin or watery tears. An estimated 10 to 20 percent of the population has some combination of these symptoms. Extreme dry eye symptoms can be serious, producing pain and, if ignored, blindness in the most extreme cases.

People who have had LASIK surgery have a greater risk for developing this complication than do people who have had PRK. In fact, dry eye is one of the most frequent complications after LASIK surgery. As many as seven out of ten people undergoing the procedure experience its irritating effects, including itchiness, burning, eyelid stickiness, and stinging. Treatment to ease its symptoms can last more than six months following surgery.

Dry eye syndrome has more than one cause. The different conditions, which produce the same symptoms, are referred to collectively as tear film abnormalities. If your physician knows or recognizes that you have a tear film abnormality *before* you have LASIK surgery, you can still have a successful result *providing* your condition is treated before the laser touches your eye.

Did You Have Dry Eyes before Surgery?

If your eyes feel itchy or burning, or if you experience crusty eyelids, tearing (especially when using the computer or when reading), light sensitivity, a sensation of grit or sand in your eye when nothing is there, redness, a feeling of pressure, or if wind hurts your eyes and makes you tear more, you probably have a problem with a tear-film abnormality or dry eye.

If you were not tolerating your contact lenses as well as you had in the past, and you found yourself using rewetting drops more frequently, you probably had dry eyes before your surgery. Some people choose to have LASIK surgery because of these problems. This is an excellent example of the importance of communication between doctor and patient. It is crucial that you tell your doctor about such problems before you agree to surgery.

Causes of Dry Eye Syndrome

Several common problems can cause you to suffer from the symptoms of dry eye. These include an inability to form the watery part of the tears (true dry eye or aqueous-deficient dry eye, which is traced to a problem with the tear-producing lacrimal glands), too rapid evaporation of the tear film coating the eye (tear film instability or evaporative dry eye, which can be traced to problems with the oil-producing meibomian glands), and chronic eyelid inflammation/low-grade infection (blepharitis). Each of these conditions can occur by itself, or it can be a symptom of other ailments, such as Sjögren's syndrome, a rheumatoid-arthritis-like disease causing dry eye and dry mouth.

Eye Makeup Can Aggravate Dry Eyes

The oil glands (or meibomian glands) are located in the upper and lower eyelids, where the eyelash follicles are located. Cosmetics applied around the eyes, including moisturizers, mascara, etc., can clog these glands, preventing them from secreting the oil that is essential for maintaining a normal, healthy protective layer of tears. When the oil in the gland backs up, and the glands become inflamed, the condition is called a chalazion or hordeolum. Frequent use of makeup that isn't removed properly or is applied too close to the oil glands can produce inflammation. Many ophthalmologists often see a layer of skin moisturizer on the tears themselves, a situation that is also capable of causing inflammation. Your doctor may ask you to stop using eye makeup either temporarily or permanently.

Age is the greatest risk factor for dry eyes and tear-film abnormalities. Makeup and skin moisturizers often make these conditions worse by plugging up the oil-secreting pores in the skin. An allergy to makeup can also make the symptoms worse.

Sjögren's syndrome is a major cause of true dry eye (often called keratitis sicca). If you have Sjögren's, you likely suffer from dry mouth as well as dry eye. The glands that produce tears and the glands that produce saliva are the same type of glands. And both, unfortunately, are inflamed and destroyed in Sjögren's disease.

People with thyroid disease often have dry eyes, too. The symptoms are seen in people with underactive and overactive thyroids. An overactive thyroid can cause the eyes to bulge. This increases their exposure to air, resulting in the typical symptoms of dry eyes.

Tear-film abnormalities also show up in people on very low-fat diets and in people with certain skin diseases, such as acne rosacea. Many medicines can reduce the volume of tears in your eyes, especially antihistamines and decongestants, certain antidepressants, diuretics, sleeping pills, birth control pills, certain antiacne medications, codeine, and morphine-type pain relievers.

Winter is especially a bad time for dry eyes. When homes are heated without humidifiers, increased evaporation of fluid from the eye's surface leads to the usual complaint of dry eyes.

Types of Tear-Film Abnormality

The tear film should always cover the cornea to protect it from dryness and infection. Tears also wash away debris that gets into the eye. A normal tear film has three layers covering the surface of your eye. The outermost layer is oily, the middle layer is watery, and the innermost layer is mucus.

Lipid Layer Abnormality and Its Treatment

The first, oily layer is secreted by tiny glands that sit in the eyelids around the eyelashes. The oil helps prevent the watery layer beneath it from evaporating. It also contributes to the focusing power of the cornea and prevents the watery part of the tears from inflaming the eyelids.

It's easy to see how disruption of the oil glands can cause increased tearing. Without the oil layer, the watery layer evaporates rapidly. The eye then churns out more tears in an attempt to compensate for the loss. Without the oil layer coating the tears, however, the eyelids can become red, sore, and irritated, and vision can decrease. If an oil gland gets stuffed up, preventing oil secretion, the result is a stye or what is referred to in medical texts as a chalazion or hordeolum.

Things to Help You Avoid Dry (or Drier) Eyes

- Apply makeup to your eyelids carefully, knowing that it can clog oil glands and increase dry-eye symptoms.
- Always remove makeup as soon as you can.
- Identify and treat other medical conditions that can cause dry eye (for example: Sjögren's syndrome, thyroid disease, acne rosacea, or other skin disease).
- Try to keep the humidity in your home and workplace between 40 and 50 percent.
- Try to identify environments that make your symptoms worse, such as the home, workplace, or automobile. In addition to dry air, try to avoid moving air from fans, air conditioners,

and heaters. Determine whether dust, toxins, or allergy-inducing substances are present where you work or live, and try to eliminate them.

- Avoid medications that can contribute to dry eye, such as antihistamines. Ask your doctor if substitute medications are available if your current prescriptions contribute to your dry-eye problem.
- Take breaks if you look at a computer or television screen for long periods of time. While staring at what's in front of you, the screen, page, or highway, you may blink less than you otherwise would.
- Check with your eye doctor before using over-the-counter eyedrops to treat dry eye. They might help you, but in some cases they can make the problem worse, particularly if they contain preservatives.

Inflammation and a low-grade infection of the eyelids occur with abnormalities of the oil layer. This condition, called blepharitis, is a common reason people make an appointment with their ophthalmologist. The eyelids are usually chronically red, irritated, sore, itchy, and may be swollen shut in the mornings.

Treatments of oil-gland abnormalities include eyelid scrubbing with baby shampoo, routine hot compresses, and antibiotic-steroid drops or ointment. Acne rosacea, a skin disease with the symptoms of adult acne and flushing of the cheeks and nose, affects oil glands. Treatment with one of the tetracycline antibiotics is often the key to relieving the symptoms. Some eye lubricants that have an oil layer in them can be helpful, but they also have the potential drawback of temporarily blurring your vision.

Aqueous Layer Abnormality and Its Treatment

The watery part of the tear layer is produced by lacrimal glands located in the upper, outer corners of each eye socket. It supplies oxygen to the cornea, protects the cornea from dryness, and contains enzymes and other biochemicals that kill bacteria. After spending some time on the eye's surface, this watery portion of your tears drains out through small holes in the inner corners of the upper and lower eyelids and eventually into the nose and throat. That is why we sniffle when we cry or tear. And when nerves in the cornea are irritated by dryness or a scratch, they signal the lacrimal glands to produce more tears.

As we age, we tend to produce less of the watery layer. Rheumatic diseases such as Sjögren's syndrome dramatically reduce the watery layer by causing inflammation and destruction of the lacrimal gland. Use of artificial tears is one way to try to compensate for loss of the watery layer, but, without the evaporation-retarding oil layer, they don't last very long. The prescription eyedrop Restasis (topical cyclosporine A) has been effective in revitalizing the lacrimal gland and inducing it to produce tears again. It eases inflammation of the eye's surface, a condition that makes dry eye syndrome worse.

Plugging the tear outlet drains using punctal plugs or permanently closing one or both of the tear drains keeps the watery layer on the cornea longer. One problem with this approach, unfortunately, is that you may experience excessive tearing from the outer corners of the eye.

Problems with Contact Lenses and Tears

If, as a former contact lens wearer, you could always sense the presence of the lenses in your eye, not tolerate wearing them for more than a few hours, or were always dousing your eyes with rewetting drops for comfort, you likely had dry eye. If you chose to undergo LASIK surgery thinking these problems would not be an issue, you were wrong. Contact lens intolerance is a frequent reason for people to consider having LASIK surgery, but it should be a warning sign for both patient and surgeon. It has been said before, but it needs to be said again: Dry-eye symptoms get worse with LASIK and should be treated *before* undergoing surgery.

Preventive Treatments before LASIK Surgery

Your surgeon should realize that you have dry eye syndrome before LASIK surgery and begin treatment in preparation for it. Also help your doctor help you by telling him all your eye problems. If you started treatment for dry eyes before surgery, it is possible to have minimal or no symptoms afterward. Treatments included frequent artificial teardrops, prescription Restasis (to help stimulate tear production), hot compresses and eyelid scrubbing, steroid/antibiotic drops or ointment, tetracycline pills, or plugging of the tear drains. Continue the treatments up to a few months after your surgery.

How LASIK May Contribute to Problems with Tearing

The complication most frequently associated with LASIK surgery is dry eyes. It commonly occurs during the recovery period and may last for a few weeks or up to six months. In fact, if you have a LASIK procedure, you can expect to experience mild dry eyes. In the majority of cases the symptoms are not especially troublesome and they resolve on their own. For a minority of people, however, the symptoms do not fade and they can cause considerable inconvenience. While other types of refractive surgery can also cause dry eyes, LASIK is sure to produce the condition temporarily because the procedure severs nerve fibers required for adequate tear production.

A Major Cause of Dry Eye: Damage to Nerves in the Cornea

The cornea is rich in pain and other nerve fibers. Any damage to the cornea stimulates these exquisitely sensitive sensors. That is why a small corneal-ulcer or a scratch in the cornea is so excruciatingly painful. When LASIK or PRK is performed, the nerves in the cornea are severed as the laser slices through superficial layers of the cornea and forms the flap.

The severed nerves eventually regenerate. After surgery, however, the temporary loss of information provided by the corneal nerve fibers means the eye has difficulty sensing how wet or dry it is. The feedback monitoring system—dependent on functioning nerve sensors—is disconnected. Normally the nerves sense when the eye is dry and activate a reflex mechanism that produces more tears. This reflex mechanism is disrupted with the temporary destruction of corneal nerves.

This leaves the cornea vulnerable to dryness, infection, and permanent damage. If there is already a pre-existing dry eye, it is easy to see why this situation gets worse after the nerves are cut.

As the corneal nerves grow back, they are more sensitive and may feel even more irritated than before, especially if the cornea is dry. Frequent artificial teardrops and initial antibiotics are essential to help the cornea heal.

Severe cases of dry eye following surgery have been treated with combinations of dietary supplements, such as flaxseed and omega-3 fish oils, preservative-free eyedrops, and special moisture goggles or therapeutic contact lenses.

Other Damage to the Eye

Creating, flipping open, and closing a flap of tissue in the eye can rarely, under the wrong circumstances, create an opportunity for pre-existing bacteria or irritating substances to cause problems. If, for example, you have had blepharitis (described above), bacteria and inflammatory substances may find their way under the flap, where they can cause a serious infection and inflammation. If blepharitis is not treated before and after the surgery, it could cause permanent damage. Treatment with hot compresses and combination antibiotic/steroid drops is the key to avoiding problems in this situation.

If the condition is very serious, your doctor may prescribe low-dose antibiotics such as tetracycline, doxycycline, or minocycline. It is not the antibiotic action of these medicines that is effective, however. It is their ability to enhance the oil-gland secretion and cut down on the eyelid inflammation. In cases of inflammation or infection under the flap, it may be necessary to lift it, rinse it and the corneal surface, and reposition it.

Treating Dry Eye after LASIK

More than 10 million people in the United States experience some degree of dry eye and, as explained above, everyone who has had LASIK surgery will experience the condition to some degree as a normal part of the healing process. The approaches used to treat dry eye following refractive eye surgery are the same as those used to treat dry eye resulting from other causes, such as aging.

Eyedrops

Everyone who has LASIK surgery receives a short-term treatment with artificial teardrops. Used very frequently—eight to ten times a day for the first few days, these drops are usually preservative free or at least contain only a gentle preservative. This feature is important, because preservatives, such as benzalkonium chloride (BAK)—while important for inhibiting bacterial growth in eyedrop bottles—damages the surface of the cornea if applied more than three to four times a day. So, artificial teardrops free of (or light on) preservatives are usually given. Depending on the severity of your dry-eye condition, steroid drops used as often as half a dozen times a day and nonsteroidal anti-inflammatory drops (such as Acular, Xibrom, Nevanac, and Voltaren Ophthalmic) are often added as well. Finally, prescription Restasis can be included to cut down on the inflammation and enhance the production of the watery layer of tears.

Plugging the Drains with Punctal Plugs

Another way to treat your dry eyes is to keep your natural tears (and the artificial tears as well) on the cornea as long as possible. You can achieve this by having the tear ducts or drains blocked with very small plugs. These plugs, made out of silicone, are usually inserted into the lower tear duct first. Later, if needed, another plug can be inserted into the upper drain.

As a test for your tolerance, your doctor first may insert collagen plugs into the ducts to determine whether or not your eyes are irritated by the presence of a foreign object inserted into your tear ducts. The collagen plugs dissolve in three to four days after insertion. The silicone plugs can be easily removed if they irritate your eye, or if you no longer need them.

If you cannot tolerate the plugs, your doctor instead may suggest permanently blocking the ducts by literally scarring them closed with a hot probe (under local anesthesia, of course). Although this sounds drastic and irreversible, it is not. It can usually be reversed with surgery. As with all contemplated surgeries, educate yourself before you sign the informed-consent form (see Chapter Two).

Other Treatments

Another option for treating dry eye is the use of omega-3 fish oil pills. This supplement has been shown to be effective in relieving dry-eye symptoms. It is a relatively prolonged treatment lasting months rather than a couple of weeks.

Certain contact lenses, such as Boston scleral lens, are also options for your consideration if you are seeking relief from severe dry eyes. This special type of contact lens fits over the white part of the eye and the cornea and maintains a layer of tears over the surface of the eye to prevent dryness.

As a last resort, a temporary procedure (called a tarsorrhaphy) can be performed on some patients. This involves surgically sewing the eyelids partly closed. This minimizes exposure of the cornea to air and helps keep the surface of the eye moistened with tears as it heals.

Chapter Four

What to Expect with PRK

Before LASIK surgery was perfected and became more popular, eye surgeons performed PRK more frequently. Today, it remains a good choice for some people with certain eye conditions. We'll describe this procedure and some possible complications associated with it to illustrate the difference between normal and abnormal recovery.

PRK involves scraping, brushing, or lasering away (surgeons call it debriding) the first or outermost layer of the cornea, the epithelium. Sometimes alcohol is used to aid the debridement and, of course, the procedure is done after anesthetic drops are applied to the surface of the eye. Then, a focused laser is used to vaporize a portion of the deeper, thicker, middle layer of the cornea to a precalculated depth. The depth of the ablation, or the amount of corneal tissue removed, determines how much of your near- or farsightedness is corrected.

In all corrective eye surgery procedures, it is essential that a minimum thickness of the middle layer of the cornea is maintained. If it isn't, there is a high risk of unstable corneal thinning. This could lead to corneal perforation in which the material beneath the cornea protrudes through it. This issue becomes important in very nearsighted people who require the removal of a lot of the middle corneal layer by laser ablation to correct their vision. In these circumstances, PRK is a safer procedure than the more-popular LASIK.

During and Immediately after PRK

Rubbing away the epithelial layer is very similar to having a corneal scratch or abrasion, which normally heals rapidly. If you have ever had a corneal abrasion or corneal ulcer, however, you know how painful it is and how blurry your vision becomes. Ophthalmologists often need to patch the eye to aid recovery, and they may need to prescribe painkillers. If you have been unfortunate enough to have had a large abrasion, you will remember how blurred your vision was and how it cleared up only when the cornea had healed. This is exactly what happens with the immediate postoperative recovery from PRK—pain and blurred vision. The pain, which is worst in the first two days after surgery, can sometimes be severe and require oral narcotic pain relievers.

Some surgeons start patients on antibiotic drops a few days *before* surgery to protect the eyes from infection. Immediately after the laser is used, antibiotic, steroid, and sometimes nonsteroidal anti-inflammatory drops (equivalent to ibuprofen) are added. Sometimes surgeons wash the cornea with cold saline to try to decrease postoperative pain. Anesthetic eyedrops are occasionally given for a few days to control pain. The patient is fitted with bandage contact lenses or an eye patch until the epithelial layer grows back. This typically takes three to four days. The epithelium is the only corneal layer that can grow back.

The First Week after PRK

The two main complications to watch out for during this phase of recovery are infection and abnormal or slow epithelial healing. The most important thing you can do is to monitor the level of pain. If the pain is intolerable after two days and/or light hurts your eyes, let your surgeon know right away. Pain, light sensitivity, and continued blurry vision could be the result of slow epithelial healing, a corneal ulcer, a corneal perforation or melting, or an infection called bacterial keratitis. If your vision hasn't improved from the level it was immediately following your surgery, you should tell your doctor.

Depending on how the epithelial layer of your cornea heals, you should feel much less pain two to three days after surgery. Your blurred vision should begin to improve, but your sight will still be far from perfect. Once the epithelial layer has healed well, your surgeon removes the bandage contact lens, and she may tell you to stop using the antibiotic and anesthetic drops. Anesthetic drops should never be used for more than two to three days. If used longer than that, the anesthetic itself can begin to damage the cornea.

The First Weeks following PRK

The intermediate period of healing typically lasts between a few weeks and two to three months. During this time, use of steroid eyedrops is tapered off. Your vision should steadily improve during this period as the epithelium heals further and the corneal haze clears. Healing after nearsighted correction is faster than healing after farsighted correction because less corneal tissue is affected by surgical correction for nearsightedness. If, however, you were farsighted before surgery, you may actually have worse vision than your best-corrected presurgical vision for two weeks or a month after surgery. This is due to the greater area of corneal tissue that was removed to correct your farsightedness.

A variety of complications can occur during this period of recovery. Blurred vision, as well as ghosting of images and double or triple vision, are the result of irregularities, called central islands, in the treated cornea. These irregularities are areas of raised corneal tissue that the procedure failed to sculpt smoothly and properly.

Multiple factors can result in glare and halos. If an abnormal increase in eye pressure results from use of the steroid drops, you may feel eye pain or headache, halos and blurred vision, and occasional nausea and vomiting.

Another complication from this type of surgery is dry eye. It produces sandy, gritty sensations in the eye. Dry eye symptoms can sometimes include pain and light sensitivity. This condition reveals itself a week or two after surgery and may persist for many months or even years after. As discussed in the next section and in the chapter on dry eyes, people who undergo PRK usually are at less risk for dry eye symptoms than people undergoing LASIK. If you have these symptoms, tell your doctor. Your ophthalmologist may add artificial teardrops or medicated drops (Restasis). You may also have the option of getting punctal plugs inserted to prevent excessive drainage of the natural tears your eye produces. Your doctor may also suggest you take a fish oil supplement, providing omega-3 fatty acids, vitamins, and flaxseed oil supplement.

Six Months after PRK

At this point, your eyes should have fully healed and your vision stabilized. You should no longer be taking eyedrops or, at most, you should be at the end of the tapering-off phase of steroid eyedrops. You should be happy with your uncorrected distance vision and require no distance glasses (if that is what you were told to expect). Your eyes should be comfortable, and you should have equally good vision during the day or night with no glare or halos.

Visual aberrations or distortions following LASIK or PRK are common and usually temporary. They range from simple decreased vision and sparkles or flare starbursts around lights, to disabling nighttime halos and glare, or double or multiple images seen with one eye.

Any complications at this stage probably concern the quality of your vision. If you still need distance glasses to see well, you likely are either under-corrected or overcorrected. This is the time (not before) to start discussing with your surgeon the possibility of enhancement or touch-up laser surgery. If you also see halos or have night-vision problems, sometimes a laser touch-up procedure using wave-front technology may be able to improve these higher-order optical distortions.

Chapter Five

LASIK Enhancement or Touch-Up Surgery

As discussed earlier in this book, the benefits of LASIK surgery are not immediate. You may see better in just days after surgery, but your eye is still healing and the quality of your vision may fluctuate. It may take weeks for your vision to stabilize. Therefore, when evaluating your vision after LASIK, it's important to be patient. If you experience troublesome fluctuations in the quality of your vision after your refractive surgery, tell your doctor. After examining you to make sure your symptoms are not due to a complication, she may be able to offer advice or even prescribe temporary eyeglasses that could help you with your vision during periods of adjustment.

Estimates of how many LASIK patients require enhancement surgery vary. It may be safe to say that between 5 and 16 percent of people who undergo LASIK may need an enhancement to get the most benefit from their surgery, either to achieve better visual acuity or to treat a complication. Some studies suggest that factors influencing the likelihood of needing an enhancement include age (middle-aged patients may be more likely to require a touch-up than younger patients) and farsightedness. It is also possible that people whose vision requires greater amounts of correction may need more touch-up surgery than others.

Common Reasons for Touch-Up Surgery

LASIK works for the majority of people who choose to have it done, but it is not uncommon for regression or under-correction to occur after refractive corneal surgery. This does not necessarily imply a complication; it can simply be part of the normal corneal healing process. Be aware there is a chance you will need a second operation to obtain the best results possible with LASIK. A second procedure may even be included in the price of the first. Before your first surgery, make sure you know if a second procedure will cost more.

If your vision is still blurry after three months or so, you should discuss with your ophthalmologist the potential benefits for you of a LASIK enhancement as a follow-up procedure. It is often possible to do a touch-up procedure, months after the first procedure, that corrects the remaining degree of refractive error.

You may find that your first LASIK procedure left your vision under-corrected, a situation analogous to having prescription glasses that are too weak to correct your vision. It is possible for your ophthalmologist to lift the flap created the first time and use a laser to adjust your cornea a bit more. This can only be done if enough corneal tissue is present following your first operation. There must be enough so that additional laser treatment does not leave it so thin that the structure of your eye is compromised.

Another common reason to have touch-up surgery is to correct changes in the quality of your vision that occur with time. If you never had LASIK surgery and chose to wear glasses instead, your eyeglass prescription can change over time. It is not unusual for you to need a new prescription for your glasses. The same thing can happen if you have LASIK surgery—years later your eyes change, and the laser-induced modification of your cornea no longer corrects your vision to the degree that it did. You could consider a LASIK enhancement in this case.

In other cases, excellent or adequate eyesight initially provided by LASIK surgery can fade or regress much too soon. This may also be improved with a surgical enhancement.

Some refractive errors resulting from inadequate healing of the cornea following LASIK can be corrected by an enhancement as well. Touch-up surgery may also be necessary to correct other complications of corrective eye surgery, such as the persistence of halos.

LASIK the Second Time Around

Before your touch-up surgery, your surgeon examines your cornea just as he did before your first operation. The surgeon measures the thickness of your cornea to make sure enough tissue will remain after the second laser treatment to keep your cornea strong and healthy.

If your cornea is thick enough and other measurements indicate you are still a good candidate for a LASIK enhancement, the procedure can begin. One difference this time is the manner in which your surgeon accesses your cornea. There is no need to create a corneal flap as there was the first time. Using special implements, your surgeon lifts the flap created during the first procedure. The flap can always be lifted—sometimes years after the first surgery. This process is easier than creating a flap where none previously existed, so it can be done fairly quickly.

Once the flap is lifted, the same type of laser used during the first surgery is used to remodel the surface of the cornea again. This time, however, the amount of reshaping required to adjust your vision is less than the first time. If everything goes well, the touch-up operation will be easier and faster than the original procedure.

The recovery period after your LASIK enhancement surgery is the same as the recovery period after your initial treatment. Take the same precautions you did after your first operation, and follow your doctor's instructions. It is unusual for a person to require more than one enhancement surgery, but it is a possibility in exceptional cases.

LASIK Enhancement following Other Eye Operations

The terms "LASIK enhancement" or "touch-up surgery" are often equated with a sequence of two LASIK procedures performed back-to-back. But LASIK surgery can also be used to improve the effects of other types of eye surgery. Touching up vision after glaucoma surgery with a LASIK procedure is one example. And as mentioned in Chapter Nine, in some cases LASIK may refine or touch up the visual improvements provided by clear lens extraction and intraocular lens implants.

Just as LASIK can be combined with lens implants to further improve vision, other types of refractive surgery procedures may be used to do the same. PRK, described in Chapter Four, can replace LASIK in the right circumstances.

Potential Complications of Enhancement Surgery

Touch-up LASIK surgery is still LASIK surgery. While LASIK enhancement often corrects or improves the results of an earlier LASIK or other type of refractive procedure, it is not guaranteed to do so. It also carries similar risks, however small they normally are.

Because the epithelial layer of cells covering the cornea is disturbed for a second time in LASIK enhancement surgery, the chance of damage is greater. This in turn raises the risk of some epithelial cells slipping under the corneal flap. If these cells don't grow and divide there, they pose no problem, but if their numbers increase, they can cloud vision. Your surgeon can eliminate epithelial ingrowth, but it requires lifting the flap once more and removing the cells.

Although creating a corneal flap from scratch is not necessary, the enhancement procedure still entails a flap. This means there is a chance of corneal flap complications as described in Chapter Two. Wrinkles or folds in the flap, although rare, can lead to overproduction of tears, perhaps swelling, and, in the worst-case scenario, an infection.

Even though an enhancement procedure often is done to adjust an under-correction in your vision, there is a small chance the procedure could leave you with a different but related problem: overcorrection. Overcorrection happens if the laser removes too much corneal tissue. It is also possible, though again unlikely, that you could be left with a residual under-correction, which may require another surgery. Over-correction is not so easy to reverse, because it is not possible to replace cornea substance once it is removed. You may have to go back to wearing glasses to correct this problem in the unlikely event it affects you.

Another potential complication of both first-time LASIK and LASIK enhancement surgery is astigmatism, caused by the uneven removal of corneal tissue. This too may be corrected by further surgery.

Chapter Six

Can Therapeutic Contact Lenses Help You?

For decades, contact lenses have proven their usefulness and convenience in correcting common visual problems while providing freedom from eyeglasses. Contact lenses work well for people with healthy corneas and uncomplicated near- or farsightedness. But traditional, standard contact lenses can rarely compensate for or correct problems resulting from eye surgery, even if your postsurgical vision is a perfect 20/20. Therapeutic contact lenses may be helpful. If you have persistent, serious problems with double images, glare, halos, and starbursts, and/or you experience poor night vision or other high-order aberrations, a custom-made, therapeutic contact lens may be able to relieve some of your symptoms. They don't work for everyone with complications after surgery, but they are an option worth your consideration.

The best treatment for postsurgical complications depend on your medical history and the exact nature of your complaint. In some cases, additional surgery can help, particularly if the first operation resulted in an under-correction of a refractive problem. If surgery or other approaches are not an option for you, your doctor can choose from several types of therapeutic contacts, including rigid gas-permeable (RGP), hybrid, intralimbal, and scleral lenses that might provide some relief. Because every person's eyes are different, it may not be possible to tell beforehand which lens has the best chance of helping you. It may be necessary to try different types of lenses before you find one that relieves your symptoms and improves your vision.

One well-known advantage of traditional soft contacts is that they feel less like foreign bodies in the eye than the now-obsolete original hard contacts did. The drawback of their softness is that it allows the gel-like lens material to closely assume the rough contours of the cornea, including its damaged areas. This puts the material of the soft lens directly in contact with the damaged areas of the cornea.

Because the soft lens so closely follows the aberrations in the cornea, it is difficult to correct the visual problems created by the surgically changed cornea.

In addition to being potentially irritating to the surgical site on the cornea, this relatively tight artificial covering may also slow healing of a damaged cornea. If your cornea is dry and/or the epithelial layer is disrupted, placing a soft contact lens directly on its surface can make you feel more uncomfortable.

Sometimes a special, therapeutic contact lens, such as a postoperative scleral lens (described later in this chapter), is used to form a type of protective dome over the damaged cornea. This can protect the disrupted epithelial cell layer on the outermost surface of the cornea from the blinking of the eyelids.

Could You Benefit from Postsurgical Contact Lenses?

If the problem with your vision is due to damage to the front part of your eye, your cornea, you may be a candidate for therapeutic contacts. Problems included in this category are severe dry eye syndrome, corneal scarring from trauma or surgery, and complications following a corneal transplant or refractive eye surgery (LASIK, LASEK, PRK, Radial Keratotomy [RK]) in addition to other diseases and conditions that affect the cornea. For example, a bulging cornea, a condition called keratoconus, may benefit from special contact lenses, especially rigid gas-permeable lenses.

If you are seeking help for problems that can be traced to other parts of the eye, including the retina or the optic nerve, or if you have glaucoma or cataracts, you will not benefit from the use of these lenses. Therapeutic contacts help only if a noncorneal condition is affecting the cornea, such as in complications of filtration surgery or trabeculectomy, described in Chapter Eleven.

Leaking Blebs and Corneal Abrasions

The creation of a new hole or outlet in the top of the eyeball to relieve elevated eye pressure in glaucoma, an operation known as filtration surgery or trabeculectomy, normally results in the appearance of a fluid-filled bump on the eyeball called a bleb.

A leaking bleb is a serious complication. The bleb needs protection in order to heal successfully and stop leaking. Protection can be provided by a pressure patch or by therapeutic soft contact lenses. The location of the bleb on the surface of the eyeball determines which type of lens to use.

Another use of therapeutic soft contact lenses is to comfort and protect your eye. Like leaking blebs, corneal abrasions can be treated with pressure patches or with a type of therapeutic lens called a soft bandage contact lens. This approach both protects the eye and, unlike an eye patch, allows the patient to see as well as possible while the abrasion heals.

Therapeutic contact lenses are also prescribed to treat abrasions and other problems associated with complications following refractive eye surgery, many of which are described in Chapters Two and Three. They may be used to treat visual problems resulting from improperly healed corneal flaps, dryness, striae, central islands, combinations of the above, or other corneal complications.

Orthokeratology: A Potential Solution for Problems with Glare and Halos

Temporarily reshaping the surface of the cornea to achieve better vision is called orthokeratology. Specially designed contact lenses—a type of rigid gas-permeable contact—worn while sleeping can allow some people to see better without lenses during the following day. The overnight pressure of the lens on the cornea temporarily reshapes its surface to provide better vision. A few people with good visual acuity following refractive surgery, but with annoying or troubling complications, might benefit from this approach. If the cause of their complaints, such as glare, halos, or other higher-order aberrations, can be traced to problems on the surface of the cornea, it may be possible to temporarily reshape the corneal surface in order to gain a measure of relief. It does not work for everyone, of course, as explained more fully in Chapter Nine. The cause of the visual aberrations you see and the condition of your cornea may eliminate this treatment from your list of options. Ask your eye care professional whether it might help you.

GASH after LASIK and Other Eye Surgeries

Among people who have complaints following their refractive eye surgery, GASH (glare, astigmatism, starbursts, and halos) comes up again and again. These symptoms can range from distracting to incapacitating. Because they are worse when the pupil is large, these symptoms are particularly troublesome at night, making driving a vehicle after dark difficult or impossible.

GASH symptoms can occur when the area of the cornea that was reshaped by the laser does not accurately match up with the pupil. Special lenses called rigid gas-permeable contacts and hybrid lenses, discussed later in this chapter, may be helpful in lessening the severity of GASH symptoms.

Contacts for Severe Dry Eyes

Dry eyes following refractive eye surgery can often be treated with artificial tears or punctal plugs, as discussed in Chapter Three. Some patients, however, experience more severe cases of dry eye. On rare occasions, this is a result of refractive surgery. More often, it can be traced to a problem with the immune system. In these cases, artificial tears can be supplemented with anti-inflammatory and/or other types of eyedrops.

If the dryness damages the cells on the surface of the cornea, a bandage contact lens and continued use of eyedrops may be necessary. Another option is to bathe the cornea in a fluid held in place with a special type of therapeutic lens called a scleral contact, as described later in this chapter.

Special Fittings, Time and Money

Although standard contact lenses work well for many people without postsurgical complications, they do not take into account the fact that each eye is unique, like a fingerprint. Every cornea has its own ridges, irregularities, and other surface characteristics. After surgery, the irregularities may become even greater. Obviously, the distinguishing surface features, large and small, of an individual cornea can have a significant effect on images formed by the light passing through it.

Today it is possible to accurately map your cornea using a laser beam to remotely explore and sense the corneal surface. An instrument such as a wave-front aberrometer or corneal topographer captures the topography of the cornea in this way. (The same technology is used to map the cornea before you have laser eye surgery.)

A wave-front aberrometer works by recording how light directed onto the retina is reflected back through the front of the eye. The path of light passing through irregularities in corneal tissue is redirected. By noting these deflections, your doctor can either fine-tune the surgery or design a therapeutic lens that may be able to compensate for your visual aberrations.

Next, sophisticated computer software converts readings from the aberrometer into a form that can be used to make custom-designed contact lenses. This process in effect creates a digital model or mold of your cornea and provides the information needed to produce a lens for your eye. The back of this unique lens is contoured to match the irregularities of your cornea. The front of the lens is designed and constructed to bend light to offset or counter the visual aberrations produced by the irregularities in your cornea.

This relatively involved process of custom fitting a therapeutic lens can take up to a week. This is significantly more time for both patient and eye care provider than a regular contact lens requires. The lens prescription may need to be adjusted to optimize your comfort and maximize your vision. And it may take longer to get used to gas-permeable lenses than regular contacts. You may have to slowly increase the amount of time you wear them until you adapt to them.

The greater amount of time required to fit special lenses, as well as the sophisticated measuring devices, computer software, and computer-aided manufacturing equipment required to custom-design and produce them, translates into greater expense. As of late 2009, the nonprofit Boston Foundation for Sight, for example, charged around $5,000 to fit one eye and $7,600 for two. The foundation fits a special lens called the Boston ocular surface prosthesis, a type of scleral lens described in the next section. Other eye care providers may charge more or less, depending on the lens.

You may have to work with your eye doctor to decide which type of therapeutic lens is best for you. Some doctors may be comfortable working with one particular type of therapeutic lens, while others can offer you a choice. Many medical practices offer services involving special lenses, and a few specialize in this field. See Chapter Thirteen for a list of key words that might be helpful in your search for the right doctor for you.

The time and expense associated with therapeutic contacts may, depending on your medical insurance policy and your personal circumstances, cause you to dismiss them as an option for dealing with your postsurgical complication. If you have been unable to find a way to correct your vision by other means, however, investigating the potential benefits of custom-made contacts may well be worth your time and the extra expense.

Postsurgical Gas-Permeable Lenses

Unlike soft contact lenses, gas-permeable (GP) contacts are rigid while still allowing oxygen to diffuse through them to reach the cornea. Standard soft lenses mold themselves to the shape of the cornea too much to be helpful in most cases of postsurgical complications. Rigid gas-permeable (RGP) lenses, on the other hand, do not rest on the cornea; they are separated from it by a gap that fills with tears. The tears fill scratches and other aberrations on the corneal surface. The front surface of the RGP lens, which faces outward, focuses light rays on the retina.

RGP lenses can sometimes reduce visual problems, such as glare that bothers some patients after LASEK and related surgeries. They are also used to improve vision in patients who have received corneal transplants or who have developed irregular astigmatism, a potential complication of some eye surgeries.

It may not be as easy for you to adapt to RGP lenses as it is to adapt to regular soft contacts, but they are more rugged and frequently last longer. Their rigidity can make it difficult to obtain a comfortable fit even though only the edges of the lenses rest on the irregularly shaped and/or irritated postsurgical cornea. You might be able to overcome this problem with hybrid contact lenses.

Hybrid Contact Lenses

Hybrid contacts are rigid gas-permeable lenses equipped with a ring of soft material around their edges. They are therefore a hybrid product composed of two very different materials. The soft outer ring, or periphery, helps make them more comfortable to wear, since this is the part in contact with the eye. At the same time, the soft ring secures them to the eye's surface. The oxygen-permeable center of the lens covers the cornea without rubbing against the sensitive, damaged tissue. It provides the same degree of correction as regular RGP lenses.

Both the central, rigid part of the lens and the soft skirt are available in different configurations, making it easier for your doctor to find the hybrid combination that best fits your eye. The FDA approved a hybrid lens called the SynergEyes lens in 2005. It is available in different models, one of which—the SynergEyes PS—is specifically designed for use after refractive eye surgery. Another model, SynergEyesKC, is designed for people with keratoconus, a conical protrusion of the cornea.

Postsurgical Intralimbal and Scleral Lenses

Most contact lenses rest on the cornea. Full-corneal RGP lenses, also called intralimbal lenses, are large enough to cover the cornea and rest on the eye surface where the cornea merges with the white part of the eye, the sclera. This often results in greater comfort and fit for people whose corneas have been scarred and/or are in the process of healing following surgery.

Scleral lenses extend even farther than intralimbal lenses. Scleral lenses, which are custom-made, vault over the compromised postsurgical cornea and rest instead on the white part of the eye, the sclera. This means they are larger than most other contact lenses. Intralimbal contacts start at around 11 mm in diameter, while scleral lenses may be 18 mm or larger. Some versions contact the sclera just beyond the edge of the cornea, while other versions extend much farther, covering most of the visible white part of the eye.

Their large size makes them less likely to slip from your fingers when handling them, but inserting or removing them initially may be more of a challenge. Obviously, these lenses need to be permeable to air and they must let oxygen through to reach both the cornea and sclera.

As with RGP lenses, the gap between the inner surface of the lens and the front surface of the cornea is filled with fluid. The combination of a protective shell, gas permeability, and a cushioning layer of fluid allows the cornea to heal without the irritation often caused by dry air, dust, and other airborne particles. The dome over the cornea even provides physical protection against the effect of the inner eyelid during blinking. The fluid layer between the lens and the cornea may provide considerable relief from the symptoms of dry eye. And the cushioning layer of fluid under the contact can mask the visual effects created by corneal irregularities, just as with other therapeutic contacts.

If you have a weakened LASIK flap or you have incomplete healing, a scleral lens may work out best for you. Scleral lenses have been used to correct irregular astigmatism, and they provide a good option if your cornea is so irregular that it cannot support other types of contacts.

Future Developments

In some cases, all steps taken to relieve symptoms of complications from refractive and other eye surgeries fail. Some patients do not, or cannot, benefit from additional surgery, medications, or therapeutic contact lenses. Even if there appears to be no solution to your problem at this time, don't give up hope. Low-vision rehabilitation specialists can help you learn to cope with the vision you have while eye care technology and medical treatment continue to evolve and progress, potentially bringing you a solution in time.

Keep abreast of new developments in the field of ophthalmology by consulting from time to time with physicians who keep track of the latest advancements in their field. You may find a good consultant locally, or you could make an appointment at a university or teaching hospital where faculty often become aware of recent advancements and developments soon after they are introduced.

Another potentially useful activity is to keep track of clinical trials that might be relevant to your medical condition. You can find lists of ongoing and planned clinical trials at www.ClinicalTrials.gov. There is no guarantee that a trial appropriate for you will be under way or planned anytime soon, but it could be worth your time to check regularly in case such a potential opportunity appears.

Ophthalmology is the subject of continuous research. Contact lens manufacturers continue to develop special lenses designed to aid people with corneal irregularities. In the future, it is possible that wavefront technology may be able to design even better lenses for improving vision in postsurgical patients. Basic biomedical research—for example, on the potential applications of stem cells and advances in replacement and transplant procedures—may one day lead to new treatments for repairing or compensating for damaged eye tissue.

Chapter Seven

Cataract Surgery

How to Manage Minor Complications

These days when the lens in the eye becomes cloudy, it is routine to remove it and replace it with a clear, artificial lens. Unless you had a serious eye disorder before cataract surgery, you have a 98-percent chance of avoiding any troubling complications.

Initially the operation leaves you with what you might expect: slight discomfort and itchiness lasting several days. Never rub your eyes after surgery. Some crust, which can be wiped away gently by stroking the eyelid with a soft material, may be present. In a few days you should feel fine. Some complications that usually improve with medications and time are eyelid swelling, drooping eyelids and increased pressure in the eye. Under a doctor's care, these problems should resolve themselves and you should be completely healed in a couple of months.

First, Make Sure Your Doctor Knows Your Medical History

If you are otherwise in good health, you have only a 2-percent chance of developing a complication following cataract surgery, and the treatment for most complications is straightforward. Infection, inflammation, bleeding, and swelling usually can be handled routinely by your physician. If you have a prior medical condition, such as diabetes, glaucoma, macular degeneration, or other eye disease, make sure your doctor knows about it. Make sure you receive treatment for it, if needed, before proceeding with cataract surgery.

If your eye starts to turn red, you lose vision, experience pain that an over-the-counter pain medication won't relieve, or become nauseated, get to your doctor right away. Always be aware of the symptoms of retinal detachment (described in Chapter Ten) and, of course, seek medical care for symptoms of infection (discharge, pain, and blurred vision) and inflammation (tenderness of the eyeball and swelling of the eyelids).

What Is a Cataract, and What's it Like to Have One?

A cataract is a cloudy lens. Obviously, because light passes through and is focused by the lens, it must be clear in order for you to see well. If light enters a cloudy lens, it is not focused to a pinpoint; it is scattered, and your vision becomes blurry. In addition, not enough light enters the lens, which accounts for the dimness or darkness that people with cataracts experience.

It is important to realize that cataracts are painless; they are not associated with itching, burning, or dryness. If you have any of these symptoms, they will not resolve with cataract surgery. You should tell your ophthalmologist about these symptoms before you proceed with any type of surgery, including cataract surgery.

The different types of cataract are distinguished by the specific problem causing the lens clouding. People who have cataracts most often complain of blurred vision that cannot be corrected with glasses. There are other complaints and symptoms of cataracts. Each symptom can indicate what type of cataract you may have.

Some cataracts make nighttime driving very difficult, producing glare, starbursts, or halos around lights. Others leave the distance vision relatively unaffected, but greatly disrupt reading and close-up work. Yet others make you temporarily "blind" under bright-sunlight conditions.

Some cataracts slowly become denser over many years. By the time the patient realizes her vision is disrupted, the cataracts are quite mature and dense. This type of cataract tends to dim the brightness of colors as well, so blacks, blues, and browns are hard to distinguish, and the color white takes on a yellowish to brown hue. People with this variety of cataract often remark how white and vivid things appear after cataract surgery.

One patient who had painted her bathroom yellow before her surgery remarked after her operation that she hadn't realized just *how* yellow she had painted it. An early sign of this kind of lens clouding is frequent changes in prescription lenses. These patients go from needing only reading glasses to needing only distance glasses instead. In this case, the patient is becoming progressively nearsighted because of the presence of the cataracts.

If You Have Cataracts, You're Not Alone

Cataracts are the leading cause of reversible blindness and vision disruption throughout the world. It costs Medicare close to $3.5 billion each year to treat cataracts. In 2004 an estimated 2.5 million cataract surgeries were performed in the United States, and that number is expected to grow as baby boomers age.

One type of cataract grows very fast—over the course of just months. It first creates the sensation that you are looking through a frosted glass, and then it completely disrupts your vision. This type of cataract often happens after long-term steroid (prednisone) use, either in drops or pills.

Who Is at Risk?

The most frequent cause of cataracts is aging; people older than 70 years are most at risk. With aging, the natural lens becomes large enough that its normal mechanism of keeping itself clear is no longer sufficient. It starts to become cloudy and turns a shade of green to brown as it enlarges. Theoretically, if we all live long enough, we all get symptomatic cataracts.

People who have diabetes and those who are taking, or who have taken, steroid medications or drops for long periods of time are also very susceptible to this type of visual impairment. This is because the lens' environment is disrupted by biochemical factors such as high blood sugar concentrations and free radicals, factors that are associated with diabetes and use of steroid medications. Trauma can also disturb the lens' natural protected environment, as can glaucoma and surgery to correct problems with the cornea and retina.

Some types of cataracts are inherited and can occur in young people of affected families. Other forms are congenital. Even babies may be born with cataracts due to developmental disease, infection, or toxic substances in the womb.

A common belief among patients is that sun exposure is a major risk factor for cataracts. This is only partly true. The compilation of many studies indicates that ultraviolet (UV) light exposure is a risk in producing a particular type of cataract called cortical cataract. Statistically, though, UV light exposure accounts for only about 4 to 5 percent of all cataracts, a much smaller percentage than most people believe.

One thing is certain: Whatever you may have read about curative vitamins, glasses, contact lenses, eye exercises, or unheralded cures described on the Internet and in magazines or shown in TV infomercials, nothing cures cataracts short of surgery.

What Does Cataract Surgery Involve?

Cataract surgery is the most successful and most frequently performed of all surgeries in the world. Typical success rates are between 95 and 99 percent. Nevertheless, cataract removal does involve cutting into the eyeball, so it is not without risk. To understand what can go wrong with cataract surgery and to understand treatment for these complications, it helps to know some facts about the procedure itself.

Cataract surgery is very different from LASIK. Instead of reshaping the cornea with a laser, eye surgeons operate inside the eyeball itself. The natural lens is suspended from tiny muscle fibers right behind the pupil. It is enclosed in a very thin structure called the capsular bag. The front part of the capsule is only 8/10,000 inch thick, and the back is a mere 8/100,000 inch thick.

The eye is first anesthetized with either an eyedrop or a numbing injection in the eye socket, which you don't feel. Many patients also are given intravenous sedation for the duration of the operation. Then, with the aid of a microscope, the surgeon either makes a small incision in the cornea or just outside the cornea with a sharp knife. Though this cut is only 1/10 of an inch wide, it accommodates the insertion of instruments that are used to remove the cataract. After making the incision, the surgeon inserts a jelly-like material, called viscoelastic, into the front segment or anterior chamber of the eye. It keeps the chamber from collapsing during surgery by acting as a space filler.

The surgeon then opens the front part of the capsule without tearing the back part. This is a very tricky and delicate part of the operation. Through that opening, the surgeon breaks up the lens into small pieces. Contrary to what most patients believe, this is not a laser procedure. The lens is broken up using ultrasound energy in a process called phacoemulsification. Pieces of the broken lens are suctioned out of the tiny incision.

The surgeon then inserts a folded artificial lens implant into the capsule bag through the front opening. The viscoelastic space filler is removed, and the wound is tested for leakage. Much more often than not, no stitches are necessary because the wound self-seals.

The patient, wearing a shield to protect the eye, can go home a few minutes after the surgery. Typical time spent in the operating room is about 30 to 45 minutes. The exact time depends on the type of anesthesia used during the procedure.

What to Expect during Cataract Surgery

Most patients are usually seen one day, one week, one month, and then six to eight weeks after surgery. During the last visit, the final prescription for glasses can be checked. Remember, cataract surgery by itself is not designed to eliminate the need for glasses; its only goal is to remove the cloudiness or blurriness of your vision. However, premium presbyopic/multifocal lens implants are now available and are being touted for a spectacle-free post-cataract life (discussed in Chapter Eight).

You can expect to use antibiotic, steroid, and in some cases, nonsteroidal, anti-inflammatory drops for the first week after surgery. Other surgeons may have you start taking certain eyedrops (usually nonsteroidal, anti-inflammatory, and sometimes antibiotic, drops) a few days before the surgery.

Immediately after Surgery

The first few hours after surgery are spent with a plastic shield (or a patch) covering your eye. Sight in the repaired eye is blurred at this point, and you may see just light or a fog in the center part of the vision. It is similar to the afterimage you see when you glance at the sun or at a flashbulb. In fact, it *is* an afterimage. Your surgeon illuminated the operating field, your eye, with a bright light during the surgery. The bright light does no harm as long as it does not shine into your eye for more than two hours, something that would not happen even if a complication developed during the procedure.

You may experience double vision for a few hours after surgery. This typically happens if your eye has been anesthetized with a numbing injection (usually Xylocaine) that temporarily paralyzes or weakens the eye muscles. This prevents the movement of one eye from being coordinated with the movement of the other.

It is common to feel like something is in the eye. Some people swear there is a suture in the eye when there isn't. Artificial teardrops, Tylenol, and time should help.

First Week after Surgery

You should be feeling better and have no double vision the day after surgery. You should already notice that images are brighter than they were before surgery, even though your vision is still blurred. Depending on how much ultrasound energy was needed to remove your cataract—which in turn depends on how dense your cataract was—you may have some residual blurriness, but your vision should certainly be better than it was immediately after surgery.

Some patients are wowed by their sight on the first day. They may be able to see almost 20/20 at a distance with no glasses, but 20/20 one day after surgery is the exception, not the rule. Others are just as happy even though they may not see 20/20 but can see much better than before. Some cataracts blur the vision so much that you cannot even see the fingers in front of your face. In cases like that, being able to make out any letters at all on the eye chart is a great improvement.

You may continue wearing the plastic shield over your eye when you sleep so you don't rub your eye by accident. And antibiotic eye-drops are used for the first week.

This is the most critical time. It is when vision-threatening infections and inflammations are most likely to occur, if you are in that small minority. Your surgeon may ask you to closely monitor your vision in the first week and ask you to call him with any serious concerns. The feeling of having a "stitch" in your eye should be slowly fading. Most patients are able to return to driving two days after surgery. If you have been working—unless you work in a very dusty and/or dirty environment—you can probably return to work two to three days after the cataract is removed.

First Month and After

Your eyesight should get progressively better after the first week. If the implant power of the lens you received was set to correct your distance vision, then you may require reading glasses. You should be back to enjoying most of your activities by now, although your doctor might ask you to restrict your gardening and yard work, golfing, and perhaps swimming through the first month.

You'll be done with the protective eye shield, but you'll continue using steroid and nonsteroidal, anti-inflammatory eyedrops for the first month and then gradually cut back over the next month. These drops help prevent swelling of the retina, which can occur three to six weeks after surgery.

If you had prior retinal problems, such as diabetic retinopathy, macular surgery, or retinal detachment, you may be examined more closely by a retinal surgeon two months after your surgery.

Potential Complications of Cataract Surgery

Cataract surgery requires the coordinated movement of the fingers of both of the surgeon's hands in concert with the movement of both feet, one delicately controlling the microscope (usually left foot) and the other the ultrasound machine. This precise juggling act is all concentrated in an operating space of maybe 1/2 inch. Still, despite this challenge, you have only a 5-percent or lower risk of experiencing a complication. The complications that might be encountered are divided into those that occur during surgery and those that develop after surgery.

Potential Complications during Surgery

It might seem that there is nothing you can do to prevent complications from occurring during surgery. In some cases, such as those that leave you with a temporary black or bloodshot eye, this is true. But often it is not true. You can avoid many complications that occur during surgery by telling your doctor everything about your medical history before you have your procedure. Let your surgeon decide if something in your past is relevant to your pending surgery. This includes current and past illnesses and medications and supplements you are taking or have taken. An example that illustrates the importance of full disclosure is described in the following section which discusses floppy iris syndrome.

Another thing you can do to reduce your chances of complications is to keep your eyes very still during surgery and follow your surgeon's directions. Sudden movements or jerking of the eye while the surgeon's instruments are in the eye can lead to potentially disastrous consequences such as tearing of the lens capsule, dropping of the natural lens or lens implant to the back of the eye, or severe eye bleeding.

Bleeding in the Eye Socket: Any time an anesthetic is injected into the eye, it could cause bleeding. The needle could puncture a blood vessel in the eye socket (or orbit). The bleeding can stop on its own and at most leave you with a temporary black eye. The blood clot dissolves in a couple of weeks with no lasting consequences.

If, however, the hemorrhage is significant, it could put pressure on the eyeball itself, which could cause glaucoma. If this occurs, the surgeon may stop the surgery and relieve pressure in the orbit by making a relaxing surgical cut in the temple side of the eyelid. If this cut relieves the pressure on the eyeball, the surgery can continue. The small incision in the eyelid is closed with a couple of sutures.

There is a small increased risk of bleeding in the orbit when taking blood thinners. The good news is that a recent study of thousands of patients indicates there is little serious risk to your vision if you are using blood thinners at the time of cataract surgery. Some surgeons still recommend stopping blood thinners before cataract surgery.

Bleeding in the White Part of the Eye: The clear covering of the white part of the eye, the conjunctiva, is full of blood vessels. If the needle used to inject an anesthetic hits one of them, you'll see some bleeding. A broken blood vessel is a minor complication and heals in a week or two. Taking aspirin or other blood thinners may slightly increase the risk of this happening, but the damage is limited to a bruise and is a cosmetic problem more than anything.

Intraoperative floppy iris syndrome is a relatively new complication of cataract surgery, that you can help yourself avoid it. It affects people taking medications, such as Flomax or Uroxatral, which are used to treat urinary problems. They are commonly prescribed for men with enlarged prostates, but women are now taking these medications as well. These drugs have a side effect of making the iris very soft and floppy, so it is unable to dilate. This increased risk of complications includes posterior capsule rupture and vitreous prolapse, retained lens material, and pupil misshaping.

Think of the iris as a curtain that needs to be opened wide, stay stiff, and be held out of the way as the surgeon works on the lens behind it. If the pupil is narrow, because the iris doesn't dilate, the surgeon is not able to see where most of the cataract is. The iris gets in the way of the ultrasound tip and can be torn by it.

If you have *ever* taken any of the medications listed above—even just one time—tell your surgeon. He can anticipate and plan for possible complications, such as mechanically dilating the pupil and adjusting the ultrasound and suction power.

After-Surgery Complications

Cataract surgery is common, effective and one of the safest types of sight-restoring medical procedures performed today. It has benefited millions of people and complications are rare. In most instances, healing is relatively rapid and uneventful. Nevertheless, as with all surgery, it is important to be aware of potential complications and their symptoms so you can obtain follow-up medical care if needed.

High Eye Pressure and Its Treatment: It's not unusual for eye pressure to be higher than normal after surgery. This elevated pressure usually lasts a day or two and is perfectly treatable with either drops that lower eye pressure (that is, glaucoma drops) or a diuretic/water pill.

Several factors can account for increased eye pressure after cataract surgery. One is inflammation resulting from the surgical intrusion into the eye. It might also be a response to a small bit of viscoelastic—the temporary space filler—that was not removed after surgery. This material dissolves in a day or two and usually does not have to be removed immediately unless a large volume is left behind.

Very high eye pressure can be uncomfortable, giving you cloudy vision with halos, severe headaches, eye pain, nausea, and vomiting. If you experience these symptoms, call your surgeon right away. Left untreated high, eye pressure can result in glaucoma with loss of peripheral vision.

How to Tell an Emergency from a Less-Pressing Complication

The following are indications of a serious, complication following cataract surgery. Call your doctor right away if you have any of these symptoms:

- loss of vision
- pain not relieved by over-the-counter medicines
- flashes of light
- seeing floaters
- sudden blurry vision
- a shadow in your visual field
- a sick feeling, nausea, or vomiting

You should also see your doctor if you experience persistent coughing after cataract surgery, because it could pose a threat to the integrity of the eye that has been operated upon.

If the pressure in your eye is very high, your surgeon may let some fluid out of the eye immediately. After administering antibiotic and numbing eye-drops, he presses gently on the edge of the cataract incision. This allows a little bit of aqueous humor to seep out and thus relieve the elevated internal eye pressure. This gives you quick relief and also clears up your vision by clearing the cornea.

People who already have glaucoma or are susceptible to it (sometimes called glaucoma suspects) may be at risk for developing high eye pressures as a result of taking the steroid drops which are routinely prescribed for this type of surgery. This condition, sometimes called steroid-induced glaucoma, can be treated by taking glaucoma drops to lower eye pressure for at least as long as you're using steroid eye-drops. Your doctor may also have you stop using steroid drops sooner than normal to limit your exposure. Routine use of steroid drops sometimes reveals underlying, undiagnosed glaucoma.

Inflammation and Its Treatment: Inflammation is a common after effect of trauma, including cataract surgery. If the inflammation following your surgery is increased by pre-existing inflammation, increasing the frequency of steroid drops and sometimes adding a prednisone pill may help.

Many cataract surgeons now start their patients with anti-inflammatory eyedrops (such as Acular, Nevanac, Voltaren Ophthalmic, and Xibrom) a day or so before surgery to cut down on excessive inflammation following surgery. But if the corneal surface is disrupted, the use of these drugs may be contraindicated, because they may make the corneal surface worse and cause corneal erosions and ulcers.

Droopy Eyelid (Ptosis) and Its Treatment: The upper eyelid sometimes droops after cataract surgery, a condition called ptosis. This can happen if the thin muscle that keeps the eyelid open becomes weaker or separates from its normal attachment points. Its incidence varies between 1 and 6 percent depending on the cataract removal technique. The majority of people with this condition recover after six months. If it doesn't improve with time, a surgeon can correct the problem. Choose an oculoplastic surgeon, an ophthalmologist who specializes in eyelid repair, if you decide to have this operation.

Potential causes of and risk factors for a droopy eyelid include: pre-existing ptosis, the local anesthetic injection, the removal of the sticky, sterile drape placed around your eye before surgery, the pressure of the instrument (an eyelid speculum) used to keep the eyelids open during surgery, or simply irritation on the top of the eye that makes you want to close it. An exposed suture on the top of the eye, for example, easily can have the same effect. Obviously, if there is an exposed suture irritating the eye, its removal alone might solve the problem.

Complications Long after Surgery

If you are free of other eye disease, you have an excellent chance of recovering all of your vision following cataract surgery. If you have other problems with your eyes, treating them and getting them under control before cataract surgery is essential for avoiding complications.

Hazy Vision: Secondary Cataract and Its Treatment: Somewhere between 20 and 50 percent of people who have cataract surgery develop a condition called posterior capsule opacity (PCO). This depends on the surgery itself, the type of lens implant used, and the medical condition of the patient. It happens when the capsule, a type of membrane behind your new artificial lens, becomes hazy. The haziness is caused by epithelial cells left behind during the operation. These individual cells cannot be seen under the operating microscope, but they can grow and form a single sheet of cells over time. The result is blurry or cloudy vision. It can appear as soon as a few weeks or as late as years after a cataract is removed.

The good news is that treatment is relatively easy and does not require any cutting. Your surgeon vaporizes the unwanted layer of cells using laser energy generated from a crystal made from yttrium, aluminum, and garnet (YAG). The procedure, called a capsulotomy, takes less than a minute and can be performed in the doctor's office. The worst sensation experienced after this simple procedure is the annoyance of seeing bits of debris drifting across your field of vision. Sightings of these floaters subside in a week or sooner. Rarely, glare may be a complication after a capsulotomy.

As always, be aware of the symptoms of retinal detachment (see Chapter Ten), since a YAG laser capsulotomy may increase its occurrence from 1 in 100 cataract operations to 2 in 100. If the procedure is performed sooner than six months after cataract surgery, the risk of retinal detachment increases fourfold; the incidence of this serious side effect increases from 1 to 4 percent.

Worsening Diabetic Retinopathy and Treatment: It is important to make sure that any active issues—such as retinal disease—related to diabetes are resolved before you have cataract surgery. If you have a past history of retinal swelling or retinal bleeding, you need more frequent and close follow-up care following surgery. This helps your doctor spot and head off worsening eye problems associated with diabetes. The frequent visits include eye exams in which your pupils are dilated so the doctor can closely examine your retina.

You may take nonsteroidal anti-inflammatory eyedrops (such as Nevanac and Xibrom) for up to three months after your cataract surgery to prevent inflammatory retinal swelling. If diabetic retinal problems should worsen after cataract surgery, then appropriate treatment should not be delayed.

Swelling of the Retina and Its Treatment: The medical term for this type of swelling is cystoid macular edema. It occurs in many eye diseases, but it is frequently associated with cataract surgery. Ths usually happens between one and two months after surgery. Inflammatory cells in the retina cause blood vessels to leak fluid. This leakage of excess fluid then causes the center of the retina, the macula, to swell.

There is increased risk for cystoid macular edema if the posterior capsule was torn during surgery or if the vitreous humor, the jelly-like substance filling the back of the eyeball, becomes detached from the retina and oozes into the anterior chamber of the eye.

This blurs vision. Treatment can last for months and consists of steroid and nonsteroidal, anti-inflammatory eyedrops (Nevanac or Xibrom, for example). Sometimes an ibuprofen pill is added three times a day. Rarely, patients are asked to apply eyedrops indefinitely to prevent a recurrence. If the macular edema is very severe and does not respond to the eyedrops, you may be sent to a retinal surgeon. This specialist may either inject steroids directly into the back of the eye (the vitreous), insert a slow-releasing steroid depot (a formulation that releases medicine over time) into the vitreous (Retisert, Posurdex), or perform a vitrectomy, which involves removing the vitreous humor and cleaning out the back of the eye.

If steroid implants induce high eye pressure, one of the risks associated with them, then they may have to be removed. Rarely, emergency glaucoma surgery becomes necessary to reduce the excessively high pressure in the eye.

Did Your Cataract Surgery Make Your Macular Degeneration Worse?: Many patients ask if macular degeneration gets worse after cataract surgery. This topic is still being debated by experts. Most studies and clinical trials suggest it does not, even though there are many anecdotal accounts of people with macular degeneration and dense cataracts who report that their central vision become worse after their cataract was removed. One possible explanation is that these people become more aware of decreased central vision caused by macular degeneration because their cataract no longer dims their overall vision.

If you have macular degeneration and cataracts, your doctor has to carefully assess which is contributing more to your blurred vision. If it is the cataracts, or you feel that your peripheral vision is getting worse or dimmer, then cataract surgery is worth a try. At the very least, images would be brighter for you after the surgery. The procedure for removing cataracts is the same in a person with macular degeneration as in one without, and the same risks apply. If you have macular degeneration, it might be a good idea for you to get the opinion of a retinal specialist before your cataract surgery.

Options for Treating Double Vision: Double vision is a rare occurrence after cataract surgery. If it lingers for several weeks after surgery and is present all the time, you should definitely see your doctor. If double vision occurs even when only one eye is open, then it is likely due to dry eye, a need for glasses, or an implanted lens that is not properly centered or has become dislocated (see Chapter Eight).

If your double vision occurs only when both eyes are open at the same time, you are experiencing binocular diplopia, which is often caused by a weakness in one or more of the muscles that control eye movements. Binocular diplopia could be a residual effect from the injection of Xylocaine used to anesthetize your eye. It is unlikely, but still possible, that it could be caused by the needle itself damaging the muscle tissue.

Use of topical drop anesthesia in place of an injected anesthetic avoids the risks of the numbing anesthetic block in cataract surgery. The problem with this method of numbing the eye is the possibility that the patient's eye could move suddenly during surgery. This could cause major disasters that threaten your vision. This cataract surgery technique, called clear cornea incision, also carries a slightly increased risk of eye infection.

You have two options if you suffer from double vision due to eye muscle weakness after cataract surgery. The most preferred approach is the easiest and carries no risk to you: get glasses fitted with prisms that compensate for the muscle weakness. The drawback is that it does not eliminate the double vision. You will still see double when you take your glasses off.

The second alternative is to have eye muscle surgery to correct the weakness in your eye muscle or muscles. Obviously, surgery always carries more risk than being fitted for glasses, and it may require more than one attempt to correct the problem (see Chapter Ten).

Chapter Eight

Dealing With Major Complications of Cataract Surgery

It's important to keep the threat of complications, both serious and minor, in perspective. Cataract surgery is a very successful procedure that has brought happiness and excellent vision to millions of people around the world. Like any surgery, it is not without risk, however slight the chance of experiencing a complication may be. You may be able to decrease your individual risk for some complications of this and other forms of eye surgery if you know about them beforehand and do what you can to treat any existing diseases or health problems prior to your surgery. This includes carefully reviewing your complete medical history and then sharing it with your doctor during your first consultation.

Catastrophic In-the-Eye Bleeding

It is crucial that you follow your doctor's instructions after having any type of surgery. In the case of cataract surgery, these instructions include advice not to exert yourself by bending, straining, or lifting a heavy object too soon after going home. This helps you avoid an extremely rare disaster formally called expulsive hemorrhage; it's probably the most devastating complication that can happen with cataract, or any other, eye surgery.

It is caused by bleeding from one of the major blood vessels in the back of the retina, the choroids. When it suddenly begins to bleed into the back of the eye, it creates pressure that pushes the back contents of the eye (retina and all) forward to the front of the eye. It can, if the incision is wide enough, push all the eye contents through the incision. Obviously, this is a blinding disaster if not attended to immediately. This complication can happen during surgery, where it is treated immediately by closing the cataract incision. It also can happen after surgery if the patient induces increased eye pressure while physically straining. If it happens to you while you are out of the doctor's office or operating room, the longer you wait for treatment, the poorer the outcome, although, in general, the outcome is rather poor wherever you are when it happens.

Risk Factors and Treatment

Catastrophic in-eye bleeding has several patient-related risk factors. You can't do anything about one: age. Eighty- and 90-year-old individuals are more at risk than younger patients. Other factors out of your control are significant nearsightedness, a medical history that includes an expulsive bleed in one eye after surgery, a previous eye surgery, or an injury that results in significant eye inflammation. Blood thinners also pose a risk factor for this type of bleeding. If your doctor thinks that you are at risk for choroidal bleeding, he may have you stop taking blood thinners, if safe to do so, before cataract surgery.

You may be able to do something about some of the other risk factors. These include arteriosclerosis due to high cholesterol, high blood pressure, and uncontrolled glaucoma. High cholesterol can be treated with lifestyle changes, including diet and exercise, and with cholesterol-lowering medications, such as statins. High blood pressure may be controlled by lifestyle changes, including exercise and stress-relief techniques, such as meditation, and by the use of blood pressure medications. Glaucoma can be treated with eyedrops that reduce high eye pressure and, if necessary, with surgery.

Treatment for expulsive hemorrhage is surgical. When it occurs during surgery with an open incision, the incision is closed immediately, and the blood drained through the back of the eye to relieve the pressure. After these steps have been taken, a retinal surgeon needs to get involved very soon to clear the blood and reattach the retina if it has been detached. Even if treatment is delivered quickly, the prognosis for good vision is poor. You cannot expect 20/20 vision after this crisis, which is also known as a suprachoroidal hemorrhage.

The good news is that the risk of expulsive bleeds has been lowered significantly now that most cataract surgeries are done using small incisions. The old cataract-removing surgical technique (an extracapsular cataract extraction) required an incision that was about a quarter of the eye's circumference. It required multiple stitches. Surgeons doing this procedure routinely kept a prepared suture close at hand, ready to be used to close the eye rapidly if an expulsive hemorrhage occurred.

Choroidal Bleeding

Choroidal bleeding without extrusion of the contents of the eye is also a rare, but serious, risk with cataract and other eye surgeries. It can blur the vision permanently if not treated immediately. The same risk factors associated with expulsive hemorrhage are associated with choroidal bleeds. Sudden changes from high to low pressure, straining, heavy lifting, and bending are all risks and should be avoided. A small choroidal bleed usually resolves itself with no consequences to your vision. If it is a large bleed, however, a retinal specialist should be called to drain the blood clot and clear the vitreous from the blood. And, of course, your doctor will ask you to stop all use of blood thinners during the crisis.

Vitreous Hemorrhage

Sometimes retinal blood vessels can break and cause bleeding into the posterior eye cavity, the vitreous. This blurs vision tremendously. This type of bleeding occurs for many reasons. Eye movement and tugging of the vitreous during surgery may cause it to detach from the retina and break a small retinal blood vessel as it does.

Your risk of having a posterior vitreous detachment (PVD) increases with age. Signs that it is happening include the perception of a floater and some flashes. Sometimes vitreous hemorrhage accompanies a PVD.

On rare occasions a PVD causes a retinal tear that can develop into a retinal detachment. Normally the vitreous is firmly attached to the retina. When it pulls away, it can take part of the retina with it. If you experience a vitreous hemorrhage, your surgeon will make sure that you don't have a retinal tear or detachment by carefully examining the retinal periphery. If your retina was spared, your doctor will suggest you sleep with your head elevated as much as possible. This encourages any blood that has leaked into the eyeball to settle low in response to gravity. You will be examined often and carefully. Again, you may be asked to stop taking all blood thinners temporarily. If you just have a simple vitreous hemorrhage after cataract surgery, the vision should clear as the blood settles and gets absorbed, and you should count on a normal surgery outcome after that.

In severe diabetic retinopathy, abnormal blood vessels that are easily ruptured grow to compensate for the starving retina. If you have diabetes, a vitreous hemorrhage may mean your diabetes is getting worse. You may require extensive laser treatment.

Sight-Threatening Infection and Inflammation

The eye is most vulnerable to developing a severe (but fortunately very rare) inflammatory infection called endophthalmitis during the first week following cataract surgery.

A typical scenario is one in which a patient sees her surgeon the first day after surgery when her vision is good and her eye that was operated on feels fine. But a day or two later, her vision starts to get blurry or smeary, her eye begins to redden, and light becomes irritating or painful. This light sensitivity makes it nearly impossible for her to open her eye in brightly lit areas.

Warning: These are serious, abnormal signs. Call your surgeon immediately no matter what time of day or night it is. Your vision is at stake. Your surgeon should not ignore these symptoms and needs to see you right away!

This complication after cataract surgery occurs in one or two cases out of a thousand. It leads to permanent blindness if it is not treated immediately.

One of the authors (Dr. Shalaby) routinely provides each of his cataract patients with the warning signs of endophthalmitis one day after surgery and gives them his pager number. He has had only two cases of infectious endophthalmitis in his surgical career. Both had 20/20 vision after treatment because they knew the signs to be aware of, called him right away, and received immediate treatment.

Cataract surgeons spend a lot of time worrying about this type of infection. It is caused by bacteria that normally reside on the skin of the eyelid. If these eyelid dwellers sneak into the eyeball through the incision made to remove the cataract, they can start to grow in the internal fluid of the eye. Their presence invokes a response by the immune system. White blood cells move into the eye to beat back the bacteria. The result is a collection of dead white blood cells or pus, which can destroy the structure of the eye if not treated and removed.

The exact treatment depends on how badly your vision has been affected when the problem was caught. Your surgeon, or the retinal specialist your surgeon referred you to, takes a sample of the vitreous jelly in the back of the eye to determine the presence and type of bacteria in your eye. Treatment includes the injection of antibiotics and steroids directly into the vitreous. Taking antibiotics by mouth or even getting them injected into a vein is not effective for this condition.

If vision is so poor that you can barely see your hand in front of your face, you will probably go into surgery. You'll have a vitrectomy (removal of the vitreous) to clear away the source of the infection. You'll also receive an injection of antibiotics and steroids in the back of the eye.

Despite the seriousness of this medical emergency, if you get the proper treatment fast enough, you can do very well and even end up with 20/20 vision. But this can only happen if you spot the problem early and get to a doctor.

Endophthalmitis has been traced to contamination during surgery. Another factor that raises your risk for developing endophthalmitis is the number of bacteria you bring to the operating room. You can avoid bringing an abnormally high number of bacteria on your eyelid to your operation by having any previous, relatively mild (compared to endophthalmitis) infections such as blepharitis (discussed in Chapter Nine) or bacterial conjunctivitis, treated before your surgery.

Many studies have been conducted to determine how to prevent or lower the risk of endophthalmitis. This hasn't been easy, because the infection is so rare; systematic studies of prevention are difficult to conduct. We do know that sterile cleaning of the eye sac and eyelids in the operating room by the surgical personnel before surgery is critical.

Any ongoing eyelid infection or inflammation should be treated with antibiotic and steroid drops or ointment, and with eyelid hygiene before surgery. Injection of antibiotics into the eye after cataract surgery has been shown to reduce the risk as well. This step is still being debated, and its risks and benefits are being weighed by eye surgeons. Evidence supports using antibiotic drops a few days before cataract surgery and for a week after this reduces the growth of bacteria in the eye, which should in turn reduce the risk of endophthalmitis.

Cataract Remnants

Sometimes a bit of cataract material remains in the eye after surgery. It might have been overlooked by the surgeon, or it might have been left there intentionally because it was not safe to remove it.

Such remnants may be inconsequential and cause no harm, or they may cause severe eye inflammation and need to be surgically removed. The risk to you depends on the type of lens material left behind and its size. The outer part of the lens or cataract is called the cortex; it can dissolve by itself with no harm if it is small enough. Recent studies indicate that even large cortical pieces (if they are not obscuring the vision) can be left over long periods as long as high eye pressure and inflammation are controlled.

Bits of the inner core of the lens, the nucleus, are a different matter. They don't go away by themselves. Even a tiny piece of the inner core can cause severe inflammation and high eye pressure. It must be removed surgically.

Why does one bit of residual lens material create so little trouble and another bit create so much? The answer lies in the body's immune response to the different types of material in the fragments. Normally the proteins that make up the lens nucleus are hidden from the immune system and its antibodies because the lens is encased in a capsule. This capsule is opened during cataract surgery, exposing the lens to the bloodstream. Our normal antibodies have never seen these usually highly sequestered proteins. When they do detect them, they react as if the lens' proteins are foreign, such as a bacteria: The immune system is activated and tries to remove them.

The lens remnants are not foreign single cells, but rather chunks of tissue. This results in a severe inflammatory response that can seriously damage the eye. It is much like endophthalmitis as described previously, except the target of the immune response is different: lens material versus bacteria. The outer part of the cataract does not cause such a severe immune response as the inner part, and so is better tolerated by the body.

A remnant cataract typically occurs when the posterior capsule breaks as the cataract is being removed. If the ultrasound removal is continued after the capsule breaks, there is a very high risk that the cataract can fall to the posterior part of the eye.

Pieces of the cataract can still be removed at the time of cataract surgery if this happens. The surgeon switches the ultrasound machine from a setting used to break up cataracts to a gentler setting called vitrectomy mode. This allows the surgeon to cut and remove the remaining cataract more gently. The lens implant can then be sewn in if there isn't enough capsule support to hold it in position. If a cataract remnant should fall into the vitreous, it may not be safe for a cataract surgeon to remove it. A retinal surgeon then can step in and safely remove it by performing a vitrectomy and lensectomy, a procedure in which the vitreous and lens remnants are removed, and the vitreous is replaced with a sterile physiological salt solution.

Shifting Lens Implant

If your glasses are knocked askew, your vision is affected until they are straightened. The same thing can happen inside your eye if your new artificial lens becomes dislocated after surgery. You may know it has happened, because you begin to see double or you may actually be able to see the edge of the artificial lens.

A lens implant rarely gets dislocated. This does not happen if the lens implant is stable in the capsular bag and the bag is intact. If your head or eye receives a blow, such as from a fist or a ball—it doesn't have to be a major accident—your new intraocular lens can move to a position lower or higher than the pupil. Such trauma can tear the fibers that hold the capsular bag and lens implant, causing the lens implant to fall down or into the vitreous.

Consult your doctor promptly about this problem. If you wait too long, scar tissue may form and lock the lens into its incorrect position. If that happens, your surgeon has a harder time correcting the problem during operation. During the repair surgery, your surgeon may just set the dislocated lens back in place, sew it in place, or replace it with a different type of lens.

Retinal Detachment

One of the rare complications of cataract and other surgeries is retinal detachment. This sight-threatening emergency can occur following trauma to the eye or even spontaneously with no obvious cause. Some people have a slightly higher risk than others of the retina pulling away from the back of the eye. Having an eyeball that is longer than normal, which is the problem in nearsightedness, is one risk factor, and the risk increases a bit more when cataract surgery is performed on a very nearsighted person. This is why cataract surgeons often examine the retinas of nearsighted people very closely before surgery to look for structural abnormalities that can predispose myopic eyes to retinal detachment.

Removing a cataract raises the risk of retinal detachment slightly because the surgical manipulation causes tension on the vitreous, which can pull on the retina and tear it. The chances of this happening are greatest during the first six months following surgery. People under the age of 50 are more at risk than older patients, because older people presumably have already had a vitreous detachment. Consequently, less tension is exerted on the retina that can cause a retinal tear or detachment during cataract surgery in these older patients. Many of the detachments that occur after age 50 are asymptomatic or make their presence known only by a few floaters. The affected part of the retina frequently lies outside the main line of sight and so causes no problem.

A history of retinal detachment in the operated eye, a detachment in the other eye, or a family history of retinal detachments are all risk factors. Prophylactic laser treatment of these structural weak spots by "spot-welding" them lowers the risk of postsurgical detachments.

Retinal detachment does not hurt. The visual symptoms experienced during the early stages of this process, however, can help you save your sight if you recognize them and seek medical help immediately.

Urgent Warning Signs of Retinal Detachment

Here are a few retinal detachment warning signs that you should be alert for:

- A sudden, sharp increase in floaters: thin, long, and/or round bits of material drifting through your visual field.
- The sudden onset of blurry vision.
- Streaks or flashes of light in one or both eyes, a sign that light-sensing cells are firing abnormally in response to damage to the retina. These flashes or arcs of light last for a split second.
- The loss of part of your visual field, as if a partial shadow has fallen over the part of your eye that detects light.

Don't delay in getting to a doctor. Don't wait to see if the symptoms go away by themselves. They may subside for a time, but the retina can still eventually become detached to such an extent that it cannot be repaired. In that case, blindness can result.

The retina is normally attached to the inner surface of the eyeball's white shell, a layer of the eye called the choroid. The retina consists of special sensory cells that respond to light and send signals to the brain, where images are processed and recognized. The jelly-like vitreous material fills the rear chamber of the eye and is attached to the retina. Often, as we age, the gel liquefies and degenerates into clumps, causing what we perceive as floaters. If one part of the vitreous is liquid and another part is still jelly-like, then the vitreous jiggles as the eye moves. Any forceful pulling on the vitreous can separate it from the retina. The separating vitreous can also pull a piece of retina away with it. This retinal tear allows the fluid part of the vitreous to pass between the retina and the layer beneath it, the choroid, further separating the two.

Treatment for a Detached Retina

Detached retinas are treated surgically with about a 90-percent success rate. A tear at the edge of the retina with no detachment can be treated relatively simply with a procedure called laser retinopexy. The heat from the laser creates a small scar that binds the retina tightly to the layer beneath it, preventing any detachment. This procedure comes with minimal discomfort, and it can be done in the doctor's office.

Treating a retina that has separated from its backing is more involved and must be done in an operating room. Patients are sedated, and nerves around the eyes are numbed. The surgeon may inject a gas into the rear chamber of the eye to push the detached retina back against the inner wall of the eyeball. The pressure provided by the gas pushes the retina back into its proper position, where it can re-adhere. Then, the surgeon may insert rubber-band-like belts (called sclera buckles) around the outside of the eyeball. These squeeze the outside of the eye, changing its shape slightly to encourage proper reattachment of the retina.

If the detachment is small and not too far away from its normal point of attachment, sometimes just the gas is injected. Any tears are then "welded" down by laser. In other situations, a combination of the gas-bubble injection and buckles may be used.

When gas is used, the patient must keep her head positioned face-down for a few days to a week to ensure that the gas bubble presses up against the area of the detachment. This requires motivation and is not particularly comfortable.

Postsurgical treatment includes antibiotic and steroid drops. Narcotic pain killers may be needed the first week following insertion of sclera buckles. The buckles, of course, elongate the eyeball, making you significantly nearsighted. You may need distance glasses.

Vision after retinal detachment depends on several variables. The most important is the extent and location of the detachment. If the macula, the center of the retinal visual apparatus, was detached, your vision has a greater chance of being permanently affected. If the macula was detached for more than three or four days, then the visual outcome is not as good as it would be if it had been detached for a shorter period.

A detachment involving only the periphery of the retina, sparing the macula, has a much better chance of a positive outcome. There is a very good chance of recovering excellent vision in this situation.

Corneal Clouding

Most, if not all, of the corneal complications of cataract surgery involve the innermost layers of the cornea called the endothelium and Descemet's membrane. The endothelium keeps fluid inside of the eye from entering the inner layers of the cornea and consequently clouding them. We were all born with a finite number of cells in this proactive layer (the endothelium) of the cornea. As we age, the cells degenerate and are not replaced. Most of us were born with more than enough spare cells in this layer—enough to keep the cornea clear throughout our lifetime.

Some people with an inherited disease called Fuchs' corneal dystrophy, however, are born with fewer spare cells in the endothelium of the cornea than normal. As these people age, a number of cells die off, and they eventually reach a critical number below which the endothelium cannot protect the cornea. Exposed to fluid from the inner eye, their corneas begin to get cloudy.

When the cornea becomes cloudy, vision is severely impaired and glare can be a major problem as well. People with early Fuchs' changes are very susceptible to losing more of these critical cells and can tip over to severe corneal clouding requiring transplant surgery. Fortunately, ophthalmologists can see the beginning of Fuchs' dystrophy even before the cornea is cloudy. If you are showing signs of this condition, your doctor may recommend a high-salt eyedrop called Muro-128. It helps keep the cornea clear by acting as a chemical astringent, sucking fluid from the cornea.

The application of ultrasound energy and the surgical manipulation done just underneath the cornea during cataract surgery can cause some of the endothelial cells to degenerate. This happens in everyone, including people who have not inherited Fuchs' corneal dystrophy. As explained earlier, most of us have enough spare protective corneal cells, so we don't notice the loss.

If your endothelium cell count is borderline, however, the cataract surgery may tip you over to cloudiness within weeks to months. This is why surgeons use certain techniques to attempt to protect the cornea during cataract surgery. These include using a protective coating for the cornea during surgery (viscoelastics) and minimizing the ultrasound energy used to break up the cataract.

Sometimes, if the cataract is particularly dense, an older surgical method for removing cataracts—one that does not use ultrasound energy—is a better option. If your medical history and condition convince the surgeon that your cornea has a high risk of failing after cataract surgery, she may recommend a combined simultaneous or sequential cataract extraction and corneal transplant procedure.

Occasionally, even without Fuchs' dystrophy, a cornea can fail after cataract surgery, especially if the cataract was very dense and required lots of ultrasound energy to break it up and remove it. A 30- or 60-day regimen of Muro-128 eyedrops right after the cataract surgery may be all that is needed to prevent this from occurring.

Other risk factors for corneal clouding include a leftover nuclear cataract, the vitreous touching the cornea, and certain (old model) lens implants.

Chapter Nine

Intraocular Lens Implants and Refractive Surgery for Presbyopia

The flexibility of the lens of the human eye is what gives it the ability to adjust its shape to focus on nearby objects. However, as early as age 12, the lens slowly starts to lose that flexibility. Fortunately, we don't notice its decreasing flexibility until our late 30s or early 40s, when this condition—called presbyopia—finally forces us to get reading glasses. Had we evolved with arms only 4 inches long and been forced to read everything in fine print, we would notice the change before middle age. Or, if we had evolved arms 4 feet long and routinely read an 18-point font, we would start complaining much later in life.

One strategy for overcoming this natural process is called monovision, an optical approach that creates a visual division of labor. Your dominant eye is optimized to see objects far away and your other eye is optimized to see objects up close. Monovision can be achieved with the help of clear lens extraction (the replacement of your natural lens with an artificial one), corneal reshaping using conductive keratoplasty (CK), contact lenses, or LASIK.

Refractive Clear Lens Extraction

LASIK surgery is an option for achieving monovision if you don't like to, or can't, wear contact lenses. This can be done with LASIK by reshaping the cornea to induce nearsightedness in your nondominant, "reading" eye. But LASIK's ability to correct bad cases of near- or farsightedness has limits. In the early days of LASIK surgery, the laser machines were the limiting factors. Today, the amount of corneal tissue that can be safely removed by the laser, or the amount that is left after surgery without causing corneal instability, are the limiting factors. This is why very nearsighted people are not good candidates for LASIK. It would not be safe, because much of their corneas would have to be removed to compensate for their extreme myopia.

Glaucoma, a history of herpes corneal disease, and other conditions affecting the cornea also may make you a poor candidate for LASIK. If you are still interested in getting rid of your eyeglasses, you can ask your doctor about a procedure that basically amounts to cataract surgery without the cataract.

Refractive clear lens extraction replaces your natural lens with an artificial lens chosen for its improved focusing ability. It is just like having cataract surgery, except for the fact that your lens does not have a cataract and is being replaced with a lens implant for cosmetic (refractive) purposes only. Your surgeon can choose from a variety of lens implants that come in a wide range of strengths.

Complications of clear lens extraction are quite different from those associated with LASIK and are the same as cataract surgery. They include retained lens material, infection, inflammation, bleeding, and glaucoma. The risk of retinal detachment is especially high (up to 10 times the normal risk) in very nearsighted individuals. This is an important point, because clear lens extraction is often performed as an alternative to LASIK in very nearsighted individuals whose corneas are too thin to qualify them for LASIK surgery. The procedure and its complications are the same as those described in Chapters Seven and Eight.

Clear lens extraction has its limits as well. Astigmatism, for example, may not be fully correctable using this approach. Lens implants that correct astigmatism are new and can't yet correct a very broad range of vision problems caused by the uneven curvature or asymmetry of the cornea surface that causes this condition.

The most common complication associated with lens implants to correct astigmatism is movement of the new lens during or right after surgery. If your implant shifts off its proper line or axis, you will have blurred vision and images will appear bent. This can be corrected by returning to the operating room within one week after the first surgery for a lens realignment. Another option, if necessary, is to completely replace the lens implant.

Cataract surgery itself may produce some astigmatism, depending on the surgeon's technique and the way the eye heals. The good news is that after your clear lens extraction, LASIK surgery may be able to correct the astigmatism or any leftover near- or farsightedness. The surgeon can also use what is called limbal relaxing incisions to reduce a mild amount of astigmatism. These shallow incisions of various lengths and depths are made to reduce the tension on the cornea as well as reshape it. They can be done at the time of the lens extraction.

It's important to understand that you may need reading glasses after a clear lens extraction. Most lens implants do not have the flexibility to focus well for sharp, near vision. Up until a few years ago, there was no good solution for this problem. If you were in your 20s or 30s and you received a clear lens extraction, your eyes would be like the eyes of someone in their 50s in one important sense: You would need glasses to read.

Newer, premium lens implants now have very useful, built-in optical engineering features that may allow you to see distances clearly and read most print without glasses. One implant Crystalens even has the ability to move and focus for near vision as well.

Multifocal Lens Implants

Multifocal lens implants are designed to provide good vision over a range of distances. The lens is divided into multiple, concentric circles. Each circle has a different focusing power capable of correcting near, intermediate, or distant vision, depending on the size of the pupil. For example, when you read, your pupil is smaller than it is when you look at something far away. A multifocal lens takes advantage of this physiological fact. When small, your pupil admits light mostly through the center of the lens implant, which is engineered to correct close-up vision. When enlarged, your pupil takes in much more light, which passes through outer rings that are engineered to focus distant vision. Thus, the power of the lens implant's innermost circle of focusing ability is strong enough for reading, while its outer circle lens power is right for distance vision.

Complications and Treatment Options

Older multifocal lens implants are prone to complications like halos, glare, and other distortions around lights. This is inherent in a design that uses concentric circles of lens material with different focusing power. The visual effect is highly dependent on how your pupil dilates and constricts while reading and seeing lights. If your pupil dilates midway between two circles, you will see more unwanted visual effects such as halos and glare.

Moreover, although each of the circles corrects for near, distant, or intermediate vision, the reality is a compromise on all these visual fronts. As a result, your vision may not be as sharp as it would be if each of your distant-, intermediate-, and near-vision needs were to be corrected individually.

For these reasons, your decision to have a multifocal lens implanted in your eye is not an easy one. If you want or need very sharp vision, then multifocal lenses are not for you. If you receive multifocal lenses and then see troubling glares, halos, and ghosting, your solution might be to exchange your multifocal implant for a nonmultifocal, or monofocal, lens implant. With a monofocal lens, you have to choose between close or distant vision. If your priority is to use the monofocal lens for close vision, you need glasses or contacts for seeing distance. On the other hand, if, for example, you prefer to drive with the monofocal lens and use glasses for reading, you can choose a monofocal implant that provides distant (but not close) vision.

Accommodating Lens Implants

The Crystalens is based on the most up-to-date understanding of how our lens focuses on something close. This lens is equipped with hinges at opposite ends. These moveable points of attachment allow the lens to bend forward when focusing on nearby objects. When you look into the distance, the lens assumes a shape that allows you to see images far away. The focusing ability of this lens is independent of the size of your pupil. This results in fewer complications, such as halos, glare, and ghosting.

This type of lens implant can shift, however, increasing its power and blurring your vision. A perfect cataract-type surgery is required to achieve the best vision possible with the Crystalens. Its surgical implantation requires additional, specialized training.

Other accommodating lenses are being developed but have not yet been approved by the FDA. Still experimental, some of these lenses respond to changes in the amount of light to change their lens power. Others respond to extremely small differences in temperature as the lens changes its shape to accommodate different focusing needs.

Corneal Surgical Manipulations

After LASIK surgery, the most frequently used corneal surgery for correcting a middle-aged lens' inflexibility is called conductive keratoplasty

(CK). CK changes the shape of the cornea by using heat energy applied by a small probe to the periphery of the cornea. This technique essentially shrinks the cornea and induces a small degree of nearsightedness. Its effect is like having monovision but without supplemental contact lenses or LASIK. CK is applied to the nondominant eye used for reading.

Monovision is not for everyone. Individual differences in the structure of your cornea may make you a poor candidate for CK. Complications include loss of depth perception, worsening night vision, halos, and occasionally headaches. It is best to try monovision with contact lenses before committing to surgery. The main complication of CK is loss of effect; the effect of the heat on the cornea's shape can fade in time.

Intrastromal Corneal Ring Segments

Intrastromal ring segments, manufactured under the brand names Intacs and Ferrara rings, are bits of clear, acrylic-like material similar to that used in many types of lens implants. (The FDA has approved Intacs for use in the United States. Ferrara rings are only available outside the United States as of 2010.) Shaped like a section, or arc, of a ring, they are inserted through incisions made in the periphery of the cornea. Once in place, they reshape and flatten the center of the cornea, decreasing nearsightedness. Ring segments are not an option if you are farsighted, and they don't help if you have astigmatism.

The thicker the ring segment, the more nearsightedness is reduced. One advantage associated with the procedure when it first became available was its reversibility, something that distinguished it from LASIK or clear lens extraction. It also had fewer potential side effects. And it has been suggested, at least theoretically, that ring segments may produce fewer complications from glare and halos. Nevertheless, people whose eyes dilate widely in the dark may still complain of halos.

Because stromal ring segments can only correct mild nearsightedness, they have become much less popular than LASIK. In addition, the procedure can be painful or, at least, uncomfortable. It takes longer than routine LASIK surgery, and it requires superspecialized training for the surgeon and special equipment for insertion of the rings.

Many conditions may disqualify you from intrastromal ring segments, including insulin-requiring diabetes, previous herpes infection of the eye, poor healing of the cornea, immune deficiency, and severe inflammatory eye disease.

The vast majority of recipients of intrastromal ring segments seem happy with them, but as many as 15 percent of patients become dissatisfied, because they don't improve their vision as much as they would like. The solution for this minority is to have them removed.

In clinical studies, some people (1 in 100) have lost some vision after insertion. This can result from bacterial infection (treated with strong antibiotic eyedrops), dislodgment of the implant (requiring removal of the segment), incorrect placement of the ring segments (either too shallow or too deep), or thinning of the cornea near the ring segment.

If placement is too shallow, the central part of the cornea will not flatten correctly, resulting in blurred vision. This also increases the risk of the ring segment protruding to the outside of the cornea. If placement is too deep, there is a risk of perforating the innermost segment of the cornea. This can result in a cloudy cornea and may necessitate a corneal transplant. In either case, removal of the ring segment (without attempting to replace it) is the best option.

Ring segments, like Intacs, can cause a variety of complications: astigmatism if the rings are not placed properly; dry eye due to decreased corneal nerve sensitivity (in which case, artificial tears are needed); abnormal blood-vessel growth at the insertion site, causing inflammation (treated with frequent steroid drops, which themselves increase the risk of cataracts and glaucoma); and a nonhealing corneal abrasion requiring contact lenses or frequent patching.

Irritating visual problems have occurred in up to 15 percent of patients receiving ring segments. This includes difficulty driving at night with disabling halos around lights (up to 5 percent of patients), double or triple vision in the implanted eye, and sensitivity to light. If any of these complications affects you after receiving intrastromal corneal ring segments, the most definitive solution, as always with this procedure, is to have them removed.

The best use of Intacs has been in the treatment of moderate keratoconus, a conical protrusion of the cornea, before the need for a corneal transplant. Although patients receiving this treatment still require correction, either with contact lenses or glasses, after the implant, they nevertheless enjoy significantly improved vision. This is especially important since LASIK and other laser corneal refractive surgery cannot be used to treat keratoconus. The same complications described above can occur when Intacs are used to treat keratoconus, but this is the only alternative treatment short of corneal transplants for people with this condition.

Orthokeratology

Orthokeratology is a procedure that attempts to change the shape of the cornea with rigid gas-permeable contact lenses worn overnight. The residual effect of the lenses on the corneal surface allows people to forego use of glasses or contact lenses during the day. The effect slowly wears off during the day, so you see best in the morning and worst in the evening. However, up to a third of patients who try this approach discontinue it due to discomfort and pain associated with the contact lenses worn overnight. Clinical studies have shown that it is best for mild nearsightedness (not farsightedness), and it does not correct for astigmatism. You have to be especially motivated to use orthokeratology as well as want to avoid LASIK. As with many overnight contact lenses, eye infection and corneal ulcers are a risk, which would require strong antibiotic drops. In the worst-case scenario, corneal ulcers may leave opaque scars on the cornea.

Chapter Ten

Dealing With General Complications of Eye Muscle Surgery

With two eyes located in the front of our heads (and not on the sides as in nonprimates) we humans enjoy good peripheral vision and depth perception. By moving our eyes to the left and right and up or down we see more of our environment. When both eyes are aligned properly and able to move in a well-coordinated fashion, we perceive depth because we have stereovision.

Six pairs of eye muscles move the eyes within their sockets and keep them perfectly aligned. If one eye does not have the same line of vision as its partner, depth perception is impossible. In addition to loss of depth perception, misalignment results in seeing double.

Strabismus or Cross-Eye

Misalignment or wandering of one eye, a condition called strabismus, is classified as either childhood or adult misalignment. Trauma, strokes, and muscular and neurological diseases also can result in misaligned eyes.

The six muscles that move each eye are controlled by nerves that link the individual muscles to the brain. Therefore, there can be more than one cause of crossed eyes or double vision. For example, eye muscles can become weak or too strong, or nerve damage can interfere with muscle function. Even a problem originating outside the eye, in the part of the brain that controls the nerves, can prevent proper eye alignment.

The control of eye movement is quite complicated. It requires precise coordination among muscles in one eye along with simultaneous coordination of their counterpart muscles in the opposite eye. This muscle control is coordinated by dedicated groups of nerve cells in the brain.

When your eyes are open and you gaze at something, the muscles in both eyes exert energy while contracting to keep you from seeing double. Since both eyes are normally coordinated with each other, you cannot voluntarily move one of your eyes without moving the other.

Controlling Your Eye Movement: Not as Simple as You Might Think

The control of eye movement is a sophisticated process. For example, when you look to your right, the lateral rectus muscle of your right eye has to contract. This contraction pulls the eye away from its "eyes front" position. At the same time, the medial rectus muscle of the right eye has to relax — otherwise the eye wouldn't move. This contraction-relaxation process must take place simultaneously to prevent double vision. At the same time, the medial rectus muscle of the left eye has to contract and the left lateral rectus muscle has to relax for the left eye to look toward the right. This simple action is coordinated by the brain. If your eye muscles relaxed completely, as they do in a comatose person, each eye would role upward and outward. If you could see in such a state, you would obviously see double.

During routine eye examinations, patients are asked to look to the right and left. Some patients, without joking, ask, "Which eye?" Normally, both of your eyes move in coordination; you cannot voluntarily move one eye without moving the other. We believe that only chameleons and sea horses have the ability to move their eyes independently of each other.

Cross-eye can occur in children or in adults. Usually a cross-eyed child does not see double but may fix alternately with each eye. If you develop cross-eye as an adult, you usually see double if both eyes see equally well. Often if one eye develops very poor vision as an adult, it either gradually drifts extremely out or—more rarely—in, because the brain has essentially learned to ignore the blurred vision of this eye. You do not see double, because the blurred image is so off-center that it is not even perceived by your brain. If your eyes were only slightly crossed, however, you may complain of an annoying shadow next to a clear image. People often go for cosmetic strabismus surgery to correct an extreme drift in one eye. It is important that the eyes are perfectly aligned after the surgery. Otherwise, the annoying double-shadow image appears.

Misaligned Eyes

Six pairs of eye muscles move the eyes within their sockets and keep them perfectly aligned. If one eye does not have the same line of vision as its partner, depth perception is impossible. In addition to loss of depth perception, misalignment results in seeing double.

When the Eye Turns Inward

The most common abnormal eye alignment in children involves an eye that turns toward the nose. This inward-turning eye, a condition called esotropia, accounts for more than half of all cases of strabismus. One or both of a child's eyes can turn inward due to a variety of reasons. These include very poor eyesight in one or both eyes, too-weak or too-strong eye muscles, problems with the nerves that control the muscles, a cataract, or a retinal tumor. If you notice an inward-turning eye in yourself or your child, you should seek eye care.

First, it's important to determine whether the eye is constantly turned inward or only turns inward when a child is tired or sick. It is imperative to know if the strabismus is due to an eye that sees poorly (amblyopia). If it is, your eye doctor can determine if your child needs glasses or, if there is no underlying disease, have the child wear a patch on the "good" eye to strengthen the wandering eye. Patching should begin before the eye-brain connections are hard-wired, usually by age three or four years.

Often a child is born with esotropia or develops it soon after birth. It is important to know if a child's eye misalignment is present at birth or develops later. Strabismus can be the presenting sign of an ocular tumor, retinal disease, or cataract, all of which are potentially treatable.

Warning: It can be an ominous sign if the crossed eye appears white in a photograph taken with flash illumination. This may indicate an eye tumor, such as retinoblastoma or a cataract, both of which have to be treated immediately.

Amblyopia

Nobody knows what causes most cases of congenital esotropia, and most children alternate using one eye or the other, an indication of good or equal vision. If only one eye is turned inward, then the child is likely to have poor vision in that eye, a condition called amblyopia. In this case, doctors often try putting a patch over the "good" eye to force the "bad" eye to improve its function. If the eyes have an optical error, it needs to be corrected with glasses. In fact, in many cases, glasses are all that is required. Your pediatric ophthalmologist can determine this and will prescribe corrective lenses with the appropriate strength. It is essential that the child wear the glasses all the time and follow the doctor's instructions.

In other cases, despite these treatments, an eye retains a bit of residual in-turning that needs to be corrected surgically. The earlier the surgery is done, the better the outcome. There are rare cases of in-turning where the nerve that controls the muscle that turns the eye outward is missing or not functioning (a condition called sixth-nerve palsy). If this nerve cannot efficiently control its associated muscle, then the opposing muscle, which makes the eye turn inward, is unchecked. As a result the eye turns inward.

Surgery for Eyes that Turn Inward

Eye surgeons have a choice when operating to treat esotropia: They can operate on one eye or on both eyes at the same time. Either way, their goal is to weaken the muscles that turn the eye inward or strengthen the muscles that turn the eye outward. To weaken a muscle, the surgeon detaches it from its normal point of attachment and reattaches it, using a suture, behind the original insertion point. A strengthening procedure effectively shortens the muscle by detaching it, cutting a section out of it and then reattaching the remainder of the muscle with a suture to the original attachment point. The exact amount of the adjustment to the muscle is measured with precise instruments called calipers. The measurements involve as little as 1/10 inch.

The choice of whether to operate on one or both eyes depends on the patient's vision (most surgeons prefer not to operate on the "good" eye), whether or not the patient has had previous surgery on the eyes (the success rate is better when surgery is done on an eye that has not previously been operated on), and whether or not the degree of crossing varies with the direction of gaze. The exact amount of repositioning and muscle removal depends on the amount of strabismus affecting the eye.

Before surgery: Before the surgery, precise and consistent measurements have to be taken of the extent of the misalignment or strabismus. Often several measurements are taken on different days or months to determine consistency. In an effort to determine the maximum cross that you or your child has, the strabismus surgeon may suggest special prism glasses. The surgeon compensates for the misalignment with the prism spectacles and checks to see whether the esotropia progresses and overcomes their power. Because it can be difficult to measure and treat very young and uncooperative children, doctors must often make several attempts. It also is important that the same surgeon take all the measurements, because there can be individual variations as well.

The surgery: Unlike cataract and many retinal surgeries, strabismus surgery is done under general anesthesia. Operating while the patient is unconscious is necessary because manipulating the eye muscles would be painful otherwise. Once the patient is anesthetized and prepped for sterile surgery, an incision is made in the outer, clear layer (the conjunctiva) of the eye. The muscles underneath the conjunctiva are identified and exposed. The point of origin or insertion is identified. The muscle is tagged with a suture through it, and then the insertion is cut. The muscle is then adjusted as necessary and reattached. Once the muscle is sutured in place, the conjunctiva is sutured closed. The patient is awakened and after an hour or so can go home. He or she is then examined at certain intervals after the surgery.

Surgery When the Eyes Turn Outward

Exotropia refers to the eyes being abnormally rotated outward. Like esotropia, this can occur in children or in adults. We do not understand what causes most exotropias, but they might be due to abnormal anatomy or too much or too little nerve input to the eye muscles.

Usually exotropia begins intermittently, brought on during times of fatigue or illness, and can initially be controlled with blinking or effort. This progresses toward a constant exotropia; eventually you cannot control the outward turn of your eye. Unlike children who develop exotropia early in life, most adult patients are aware of doubling of images. (Children don't see double because the brain suppresses the image from one eye.) Surgery is usually performed when the exotropia becomes constant or when the intermittent episodes become very frequent. The surgery involves the same type of surgical manipulations used to correct esotropia. Sometimes, however, eye exercises called orthoptics are recommended for certain types of small exotropias and can be successful.

Surgery When the Eyes Point Up or Down, or are Malrotated

Sometimes eye misalignments involve muscles that control vertical (up or down) eye orientation. Other conditions may involve muscles that control both vertical and horizontal eye orientation. Surgical treatment of all these misalignments is usually more complex than the procedures described previously. Sometimes surgery may involve three or four muscles simultaneously in both eyes. In other cases, sequential surgery may lead to the best solution. Complex surgery on three or four muscles simultaneously can produce results as good as those achieved with less complex surgeries, but may require more than one surgery. Strabismus surgeons, however, are always wary about operating on more than two or three muscles per eye, because it can lead to a complication called anterior ischemic syndrome in which the blood circulation in the front part of the eye is severely disrupted, potentially causing loss of vision.

Adjustable Sutures

A special suture technique has been developed to make strabismus surgery more precise. In this procedure, the muscle or muscles in need of adjustment are temporarily tied with a special knot. This knot can be adjusted more precisely after the patient has awakened from anesthesia. The procedure can be done in the office or in the recovery room. The surgeon uses prisms and other measuring instruments to determine the optimal repositioning of the muscle to achieve totally straight muscles in all directions of gaze. Once this is determined, the muscle is permanently tied with the same suture. There may be some pain with the procedure, but it has been shown to achieve more precise muscle straightening than traditional approaches.

Potential Complications of and Treatments following Eye Muscle Surgery

The balance and sophisticated nature of the nerve and muscle mechanism that coordinates movement of the eyes presents challenges for the surgeon trying to adjust it. As a result, it is not unusual for the first operation to fall short of achieving perfect results. Adjustments may be necessary. Patients may need patience before the best outcome is achieved.

Unsatisfactory Alignment/Diplopia

Despite the generally precise nature of the calculations used to determine just how much the muscles need to be adjusted to correct misalignment of the eyes, sometimes under-correction or overcorrection of the strabismus can occur following surgery. This can be caused by the healing process, formation of scar tissue over the muscles leading to decreased muscle mobility, or small errors in preparatory measurements.

Under-correction is a more frequent complication than overcorrection. Often it is corrected by a second, and sometimes a third, surgery. While this can be frustrating for patients and parents, it is an understandable necessity given the difficulty of the task of adjusting multiple eye muscles to the precise orientation. By some estimates, a child with esotropia may require an average of 2½ surgeries throughout his lifetime before proper alignment is achieved.

It is important, therefore, that you are aware of the nature of this type of surgery and the possible need for multiple surgeries. In some procedures, such as those performed to correct eyes that turn outward, surgeons make it a point to overcorrect. This causes the eyes initially to be turned inward. Then, gradually, the muscles heal and relax into the proper position. Patients having this surgery oftentimes experience diplopia, or double vision, for a few weeks following surgery until the final phase is reached. Diplopia can occur in adults and children who are around 10 years or older, if surgery results in under-correction or overcorrection.

Treatments of misalignment vary according to the cause. If you are seeing double following surgery, you might be fitted with special, temporary spectacles until a second surgery is performed. These glasses are equipped with a prism that realigns images on the retina. Sometimes these prisms can be stuck onto your regular glasses and can be removed, or their strength adjusted, as needed. These stick-on prisms, called Fresnel prisms, are relatively inexpensive and do not require adjustment of your regular glass lenses each time they are fitted. They have the disadvantage of blurring the vision somewhat, and they can get dirty very easily.

Another option is to have the prisms ground into the glass lens itself so it doesn't blur the image. This can be an expensive process, however, because it involves changing the entire lens as opposed to sticking a prism onto the surface of your old glasses. Furthermore, each time an adjustment is needed, new lenses have to be prepared.

Blurred Vision

The most frequent cause of blurred vision after muscle surgery is the development of astigmatism. This is caused by tightness or pressure produced by the altered muscle connections that realign the eye. It usually occurs when two or more muscles are operated on at the same time. The problem may be fixed by glasses that correct astigmatism. The surgeon or an optometrist should do a preoperative and postoperative check for astigmatism in young children who cannot read yet. They should correct for it, if present, or amblyopia may develop in the newly astigmatic eye.

Eye Infections

Antibiotic drops or ointment are needed for at least a week after your surgery. Sometimes infections can occur that require stronger topical or oral antibiotics. Infections can range from simple conjunctivitis to more serious conditions.

Very rarely, certain infections require emergency treatment. If you experience anything like the following symptoms, go to your surgeon or to the emergency room immediately. The seriousness of these emergencies are easily recognizable. For example, orbital cellulitis produces a red, puffy eye and eyelid, often a protruding eyeball which cannot move easily, blurred vision, eye pain, and fever. The treatment consists of intravenous antibiotics and very careful monitoring of the eye and the patient. People with poor immune systems or diabetes are more susceptible to orbital cellulitis than others.

Another infection that requires immediate emergency care is endophthalmitis, a severe infection and inflammation that occurs in the internal core of the eye, the vitreous cavity. Fortunately, it is a very rare complication after eye muscle surgery. When it does occur, it typically develops a few days after surgery and produces a rapid decrease in vision, increased redness of the eyeball (beyond that normally seen after surgery), inflammation, and sensitivity to light (photophobia). This emergency requires a retinal surgeon to sample the vitreous cavity for bacteria and inject powerful antibiotics into it. If vision is very bad (usually light perception), you may need vitreous surgery during which the affected vitreous is cleared from the eye and replaced with saline, and the vitreous cavity is injected with powerful antibiotics. The prognosis of good vision returning depends on how long you had the endophthalmitis and how bad your vision was right before treatment.

Eye Redness

You should expect eye redness after surgery, but it should clear up gradually in a few weeks. If, instead, the degree of eye redness gets worse with time, the ophthalmologist will consider a host of possible causes, including drug allergy, intolerance of the suture material, conjunctival scarring, and corneal dellen (shallow pits in the peripheral cornea that produce redness and eye irritation).

If you have an antibiotic allergy, your eye and eyelid will turn red and possibly swell. Your eye may become itchy as well. Your doctor will switch antibiotics and give you steroid drops or antiallergy drops and/or pills.

If your eye cannot tolerate the sutures used to realign it, you will notice a slightly tender, raised, red, opaque, cyst-like structure at the suture site(s) weeks after surgery. Steroid drops or ointment should treat this condition. If they don't, the sutures can be removed surgically.

If you notice redness around a pit at the border of the cornea, you may have a dellen. This is a thinning of the cornea caused by a rise in the surrounding tissue of the conjunctiva, the thin, clear, mucous membrane that covers the eye's surface. This postsurgical complication prevents adequate lubrication by tears in that area. The treatment is frequent lubrication with artificial tears and nighttime ointment. On occasion, eye patching to help the cornea heal faster may be required.

Redness also may result from scarring of the normally clear conjunctiva. If the muscle or its covering (fascia) is mistakenly sutured to the conjunctiva and then all closed together, there will be scarring and inadequate healing. This causes persistent redness or a pinkish appearance to the inner corner of the eye. More seriously, it may also restrict the eye's ability to move outward. This complication may be treated with additional surgery to free the bond between the muscle and conjunctiva.

A foreign-body sensation, the feeling that something is in your eye, may be caused by a clear, fluid-filled swelling in the conjunctiva.

This conjunctival cyst can occur weeks after muscle surgery. Topical steroid eyedrops or ointment may take care of it. If it persists, surgical removal performed during a quick office procedure may be necessary. Conjunctival cysts occur spontaneously as well and often resorb on their own.

Retinal Complications

Seeing a floater or black spot, with or without frequent flashes of light, and—more ominously—a sensation that a veil or curtain is covering part of your vision may be a sign of a retinal tear or detachment. These are rare complications that happen typically after eye muscle surgery only if the suturing needle penetrates the retina. If you have these symptoms, go to your ophthalmologist or to the nearest emergency room with an ophthalmologist on call without delay.

Your ophthalmologist may keep a close eye on a retinal tear or use a laser to create a tiny scar around the tear. The scar secures the damaged retina and keeps the tear from expanding and becoming a retinal detachment. A retinal detachment is a surgical emergency and is usually referred to a retinal surgeon for repair.

Ischemia of the Eye

Redness, eye inflammation, corneal clouding, and blurred vision may be indications of a rare but very serious complication that can occur when three or more muscles of the same eye are operated on at the same time.

Each eye muscle has arteries that are responsible for the circulation of the front segment of the eye. These arteries are disrupted during eye muscle surgery. If only one or two muscles are operated on at one time, blood continues to flow through arteries associated with the muscles that are not being operated upon. If, however, more than two muscles are operated on, there is a greater risk of interrupting this circulation. The result may be ischemia, or a stroke, to that part of the eye. If left untreated, there is a high risk of tissue death and loss of the eye.

The initial inflammation needs to be treated with frequent steroid eyedrops, or sometimes prednisone, delivered orally or injected into the eye. The best way to prevent this complication is to have multiple, successive (rather than simultaneous) surgeries on one eye. Ask your doctor about this when you discuss your impending surgery with her.

The initial inflammation needs to be treated with frequent steroid eye-drops, or sometimes prednisone, delivered orally or injected into the eye. The best way to prevent this complication is to have multiple, successive (rather than simultaneous) surgeries on one eye. Ask your doctor about this when you discuss your impending surgery with her.

Eyelid Complications

If you find that your eyelid has a different position following eye muscle surgery, additional surgery may correct the problem. This usually affects the lower eyelid more frequently than the upper eyelid.

Complications of Anesthesia

The strain of vomiting can stretch surgical sutures and disrupt them. If you experience nausea or vomiting after surgery, return to see your ophthalmologist. Eye muscle surgery, especially under general anesthesia, docs carry a high risk of this unpleasant response, which can happen as early as one to two hours after surgery and can last up to three days. This means it occurs after you have left the hospital and gone home.

It is a well-studied phenomenon that may be related to the use of anesthesia or to a combination of manipulation of the muscles affected by the surgery and stimulation of the nerves that innervate them.

Fortunately, this complication can be prevented in various ways. The most effective is intravenous administration of one of the newer antiemctic drugs, such as Zofran. Older medications, such as Reglan and Phenergan, also work, although newer antiemetics have fewer side effects. Often treatment (by mouth) may need to be continued for a day or two after the surgery.

Chapter Eleven

General Complications of Glaucoma Surgery and Corneal Transplants

The glaucomas are a group of eye diseases that result in damage to the optic nerve, which, in turn, leads to loss of peripheral vision. The highest risk factor for glaucoma is high eye pressure, which happens to be the only variable that can be controlled and treated. The goal of all current treatments is to lower eye pressure.

Glaucoma: Often, But Not Always, a Result of High Eye Pressure

As described in Chapter One, fluid is normally formed in the back of the eye and percolates to the front of the eye where it gets filtered through a structure called the trabecular meshwork. This filtering process maintains a normal range of pressure in the eye fluid. If this pressure becomes much higher than normal, it can damage the optic nerve, affect peripheral vision, and, if uncontrolled, lead to blindness. Abnormally low pressure has its own consequences, including the collapse of the front chamber of the eye.

Ballooning Pressure

You can understand the dynamics of eye pressure by thinking of the eye as a balloon with a faucet for input and a drain for output. If the input through the faucet is balanced by good drainage, then the balloon will maintain a constant internal pressure. If, however, the faucet is opened wide and overwhelms the ability of the drain to release fluid, then pressure will build up and the balloon will inflate more.

Similarly, if the faucet's input is normal, but the drain becomes clogged—but not stopped up completely—pressure will still build up because the drain is not able to release fluid as fast as the faucet admits it. A completely stopped-up drain increases the pressure in the balloon rapidly, a situation that simulates a condition called closed-angle glaucoma. Now, unlike a balloon, the eye will not inflate with increased fluid production or slow drainage, but pressure will increase.

Laser Surgery for Closed-Angle Glaucoma

Closed-angle glaucoma is a special type of glaucoma that can occur very suddenly in people at risk. People of Asian descent have a greater risk of developing it than do Caucasians. Also, people with elevated risk for this disease tend to have small eyes and wear glasses that magnify images (hyperopia).

In closed-angle glaucoma, the iris mechanically blocks the internal eye filter, the trabecular meshwork, all around the eye, so that no fluid can pass through it. This happens more often when the pupil is dilated, as in the relative darkness of a movie theater, for example. In low light, the wide pupil causes the iris to bunch up at the angle in the eye where the trabecular meshwork is located. As a result, eye pressure builds up very fast, causing eye pain, headache, nausea, and vomiting. The cornea becomes swollen and cloudy. This, in turn, blurs vision and causes the patient to sees halos around lights. When the pupil looks like it is partly dilated in an acute-angle closure, it is because it is stuck in that position.

If this condition lasts longer than a few hours, the high eye pressure will damage the optic nerve and cause permanent vision loss. Physicians who are not familiar with eyes often mistake this for an eye infection or conjunctivitis and treat it as such. Acute closed-angle glaucoma is an eye emergency and requires immediate treatment. If laser surgery cannot be done immediately, temporary measures involving the use of eyedrops and diuretic pills to lower eye pressure may help until laser surgery can be performed.

The surgery to treat this serious threat to vision is simple. Called peripheral iridotomy (PI), it is not painful and requires only topical anesthesia. Your surgeon uses light energy (from a device called a YAG laser [described in Chapter Seven], which, incidentally, is not the same kind of laser used in LASIK surgery) to make a small hole in the peripheral part of the iris, which is usually under the eyelid. The hole is a fraction of a millimeter in diameter but wide enough to let fluid out of the eye's interior. This immediately releases built-up pressure and relieves the symptoms of headache, pain, nausea, and vomiting. Blurred vision should resolve within hours once the cloudy cornea clears up. If it doesn't, then permanent optic nerve damage has probably occurred.

Once one eye has had an acute-angle closure crisis, the second eye needs a peripheral iridotomy as well, since it is at risk of developing the same condition. Fortunately, most ophthalmologists do not wait until an acute-angle closure occurs in the second eye before performing a peripheral iridotomy. With routine eye care, an ophthalmologist or optometrist monitors the angle of your trabecular meshwork for narrowness. When the doctor observes a certain critical narrowing, it is time to get a PI before an acute-angle closure crisis happens.

Complications of Peripheral Iridotomy Surgery

You may have blurred vision, see mild floaters, and be sensitive to light immediately after this procedure. These symptoms should last only a couple of hours. There also may be some mild bleeding of the iris seen as red spots. This, too, stops shortly. Your doctor may suggest that you use anti-inflammatory eyedrops for a few days to control any inflammation.

If eye pressure is not lowered, or if it increases again for some reason after the PI, then a procedure such as surgical iridotomy—in this case called iridectomy—and perhaps filtration surgery is required to control the eye pressure and prevent permanent damage.

Double vision in one eye can be a complication if the new drainage hole is not located under the eyelid. Think of the PI as a tiny pupil. If it isn't covered by your eyelid, then you effectively would have two pupils through which to see. If this happens, and it bothers you very much, the hole created during the first PI can be closed surgically, and another hole can be made under the eyelid.

Open-Angle Glaucoma Surgery

In the most common type of glaucoma, the angle formed by the iris and the cornea is not closed as it is in closed-angle glaucoma. Although the angle remains open, there is nevertheless enough resistance to fluid flowing through the filtering apparatus that pressure in the eye gradually builds up. No one knows why this resistance occurs, but it is possible to spot the condition early during a regular eye exam.

If not recognized early, the painless, gradual progression of the disease can slowly damage the optic nerve. It is possible to lose part of your vision even before you are aware you have an eye disease if you don't get regular eye exams.

Eyedrops are the first option for lowering eye pressure in open-angle glaucoma. There are many different types of eyedrops with different modes of action to choose from. If they don't work, you can't afford them, or you have trouble using them, then you should consider laser surgery. Surgery could be less expensive over the long term, depending on your insurance coverage and personal financial situation.

Laser Treatments for Open-Angle Glaucoma

Two types of laser surgery, similar in nature, are performed to treat open-angle glaucoma. Both argon laser trabeculoplasty (ALT) and selective laser trabeculoplasty (SLT), use specific wavelengths of laser energy aimed at the filtration apparatus of the trabecular meshwork. Both treatments change the filtering capacity, and possibly the chemical structure of the meshwork, resulting in increased filtration.

ALT, the older method, may be more intense and slightly more destructive to the filters than SLT. Because it uses a gentler laser, SLT may be done more than once, although the second time may be a little less effective. Both ALT and SLT reduce eye pressure by about 25 percent, which is equivalent to the efficacy of one eyedrop. However, the results of the initial treatment may not be permanent; sometimes the high eye pressure returns within two to three years. A repeat SLT laser treatment or the use of eyedrops may be useful if this happens.

The surgery itself is completely painless and typically takes less than 10 minutes. You will have blurry vision for a couple of hours after the surgery, and any mild inflammation you experience is treated with anti-inflammatory drops.

The most frequent complication, especially with ALT, is a transient rise in eye pressure one to four hours after the surgery. This can be a serious problem if you have advanced glaucoma, because it can cause more damage to your optic nerve. Most surgeons give you an additional eye-pressure–lowering medication before and right after this type of laser surgery to prevent this from happening.

If you have any signs of eye pain, redness, or halos and blurred vision, you should call your surgeon right away. If your eye pressure is indeed high, your doctor will have you use more eyedrops and/or diuretic pills until the pressure returns to normal. On rare occasions, high eye pressure may persist and require emergency filtration surgery.

Filtration Surgery

If medication and/or laser surgery do not lower eye pressure adequately, then incisional filtration surgery, or trabeculectomy, is the next choice. A large study involving multiple healthcare centers compared the effectiveness of treating glaucoma first with filtration surgery instead of eyedrops. It found that surgery did a better job at lowering eye pressure. Still, because of the risks and potential complications of filtration surgery, eyedrops are normally the choice for initial therapy.

You receive a sedative (injected through a vein) and a local anesthetic before surgery. The operation creates a new "filter" in the shape of a hole in the top of your eyeball. A triangular flap of sclera covers the hole and serves as a one-way valve, letting fluid out of your eye but not into it. The flap is secured with two or three sutures and covered with a section of conjunctiva, the thin membrane that covers the white part of your eye. From then on, the fluid from your eye will drain through the newly created hole rather than through the original filter, the trabecular meshwork. Substances called antimetabolites (mitomycin C and 5-fluorouracil) often are used to prevent the new opening from scarring or closing. The dosages and timing of antimetabolite therapy are critical, since they can determine whether the new exit point for eye fluid is under- or overactive, both of which can create complications. Also, you will take frequent steroid and antibiotic drops for six to eight weeks after surgery.

Successful trabeculectomy should leave you with a healthy eye pressure and a clear cyst on the top part of the eyeball. Do not rub that area! Often people report that they can feel some fluid draining from that part of their eye. This is normal. If you sense excessive fluid leakage, however, it may mean a problem at the surgical site, so consult your ophthalmologist.

Early Complications of Filtration Surgery

If you notice redness, haziness, or smokiness in your vision, and increased sensitivity to light, report this to your eye doctor right away. Infections, including endophthalmitis, are serious complications that can disrupt vision permanently if not treated promptly with antibiotics. By some estimates, 10 to 15 percent of patients undergoing filtration surgery may develop endophthalmitis. After a hole is created by the operation, only a very thin layer of conjunctiva separates the internal structures of the eye from external structures, such as the eyelid, where bacteria reside. Moreover, use of antimetabolites makes this layer even thinner and increases the risk of tiny rips and openings which could provide a path for bacteria to enter the eye.

Excessive leakage from the wound requires medical treatment. Again, patients are more at risk when using antimetabolites, because these substances can make the conjunctiva very fragile, leading to overfiltration and abnormally low eye pressure. In extreme cases, low eye pressure potentially could make the front part of the eye collapse. More commonly, it disrupts vision by inducing swelling in the center part of the retina, the macula.

An excessive production of tears could also be due to a leakage from the wound, which disrupts your vision. If it occurs, your ophthalmologist can increase your eye pressure by closing the wound with the aid of an eye pressure patch applied to the upper part of the eyelid, and by prescribing eyedrops. If these steps don't work, you may go back to the operating room to have the wound closed surgically.

An overfiltering trabeculectomy that is not due to a wound leak is also a serious complication that can lead to very low eye pressure (hypotony). The treatment is to enhance, rather than inhibit, wound repair. Patients recovering from filtration surgery usually use frequent steroid drops to inhibit wound repair and keep the filter unscarred and open. If the new filter is too efficient, however, the ophthalmologist decreases the frequency of the steroid drops in an attempt to get the filter to close a little bit. Sometimes the surgeon tightens the opening by suturing the filter. Injecting the patient's own serum into the eye can increase eye pressure to reach healthier levels.

Too-low eye pressure can also induce a detachment of one of the inner layers of the eye called the choroid. Choroidal detachments can produce painful headaches and lead to loss of vision if not treated. Steroid drops and/or prednisone pills can help. Surgery on the filter and serum injection also may be required.

Under-filtration is another complication that obviously has consequences for eye pressure and the long-term treatment of glaucoma. This can be both an early and late complication. When it occurs soon after surgery, it is likely due to excessive scarring in, or inadequate size of, the newly formed hole.

Most glaucoma surgeons aim for eye pressure that is slightly high. In this way, they can loosen or laser away one or all of the sutures holding the tissue flap over the filter, if necessary. When this painless office procedure is performed within the first two weeks after surgery, it should bring the pressure down to its intended target. If these procedures do not work, a needle can be inserted into the hole itself a few weeks after surgery. This procedure can clear the scarring. If this does not work, it is likely that the filter has failed, and you need another filter-forming operation or insertion of a tube filtration device, as described later in this chapter.

If you experience sudden loss of vision or see darkness in a sector of your vision, call the ophthalmologist immediately. Your symptoms may be due to bleeding following the operation. To avoid this complication, you should have been asked to stop taking all blood thinners before surgery. Choroidal hemorrhage is a very rare but visually devastating complication involving bleeding from major blood vessels behind the retina. This can detach the retina and choroid and cause sudden, severe, and permanent vision loss. Treatment includes draining the blood clot and repairing the detachment. The prognosis for return of good vision is poor. The causes of this complication include a sudden drop in eye pressure and advanced arteriosclerotic disease.

Increased eye pressure, blurred vision, and corneal clouding may indicate a less devastating complication called hyphema, which involves bleeding in the front part or anterior segment of the eye. It usually clears up over a few days or weeks. If the hyphema is very dense and is not clearing, a procedure called an anterior chamber washout is performed to clear away the blood.

Decreased vision can occur following filtration surgery. Once the complications outlined above are ruled out, the most likely reason would be surgical-induced astigmatism. The cyst on the top of the eyeball, produced by the surgery, reshapes the eyeball slightly and induces astigmatism, which can be corrected with prescription lenses.

Your ophthalmologist also has to make sure that a cataract has not started or worsened following surgery. Cataracts, which can develop within the first three months after surgery, are the most frequent complication of filtration surgery and are covered later in this chapter.

Late Complications of Filtration Surgery
Late complications include those that develop after the first three

months or so following surgery. The cyst created during the surgery should clear. If it instead appears to be filled with milky or opaque fluid, report this to your ophthalmologist promptly. You should also report smoky vision, increased redness, and light sensitivity to your doctor right away, because infection, especially endophthalmitis, remains a major risk due to the fragile conjunctiva. Wound leaks can also occur at any time, so be sure to report any increased tearing of the operated eye to your ophthalmologist. Low eye pressure is also a potential complication, and you should be sure to visit your ophthalmologist for all scheduled follow-up visits, so she can carefully monitor your eyes.

A surgically created filter can fail months after the operation, usually due to scarring and natural wound repair that closes the hole formed by the laser. In these cases, another filter is made surgically at a different location on top of the eyeball, or the doctor may perform tube shunt surgery as described in the next section.

As mentioned earlier, cataracts are a frequent complication after filtration surgery. Any eye surgery that disrupts the normal balance of the eye can cause clouding of the natural lens. If your vision is significantly impaired due to cataracts, cataract surgery with a lens implant provides the best chance of restoring your vision. A cataract surgeon must be careful to avoid surgery near the site of the hole—the trabeculectomy—otherwise, the filter can fail. Other than that precaution, cataract removal following filtration surgery is no different from a regular cataract removal.

Eyelid droop is not an infrequent complication after filtration surgery. Drooping could be a consequence of the anesthetic block before surgery, the actual surgery under the eyelid, or the presence of the cyst. If it bothers you or is cosmetically unpleasing, the positioning of your eyelids can be adjusted surgically. Sometimes an eyelid may retract at the site of the filter. This may lead to a feeling of dry eye. Artificial teardrops, preferably preservative-free, may help relieve this feeling and prevent exposure dryness of the cornea.

Tube Shunts and Implants for Treating Glaucoma

If filtration surgery does not lower high eye pressure, eye surgeons can perform another procedure that may do the job. It involves the insertion of a tube to bypass the normal filters. Fluid in the eye is then shunted to an artificial reservoir. The same procedure can be used when glaucoma results from extensive eye inflammation or when a secondary glaucoma is caused by a severe diabetic eye disease, stroke, or blood clot in the retina.

This is extensive surgery. It involves suturing a metal plate that holds a reservoir on top of the eye. A tube shunt is covered with a patch constructed from the tough, white part of the eye, the sclera, to keep it from eroding, and the tube is inserted into its proper position. The tube carries fluid from the eye's anterior chamber to the reservoir placed on the top part of the eye. The size of the reservoir determines how low the eye pressure is. The surgeon must be careful not to place the tube too close to the cornea, or else corneal clouding can occur. Similarly, the tube should not touch the natural lens because it may cause a cataract.

Complications of Tube Shunt Surgery

Many complications of tube shunt surgery are the same as those occasionally seen following filtration surgery or trabeculectomy. Specific complications include corneal swelling and clouding if the tube is too close to the cornea or has touched the cornea during surgery, and cataracts if the tube is close to, or has touched, the natural lens. Erosion through the tissue and/or migration of the plate holding the reservoir from its original position would be a serious complication requiring a return to the operating room for revision surgery to repair the damage. Newer, flexible valve devices are less likely to contribute to this complication.

The Last Resort: Laser Destruction for Uncontrolled High Eye Pressure

When all else fails and eye pressure remains too high, surgeons can resort to a laser procedure called laser cyclophotocoagulation. This last resort destroys the fluid-forming structure of the eye called the ciliary body. This procedure is performed only if you have poor vision and high eye pressure that may lead to total vision loss, or if you are blind and in constant pain from high eye pressure. It is normally performed under analgesia or heavy sedation. Its complications include continued high eye pressure, inflammation of the eye, and decreased vision. Strong pain killers may be needed following surgery.

Surgery for Secondary Glaucomas:
Complications and Treatments

Glaucoma occasionally occurs as a result of another eye disease. Typically, treating the underlying condition can resolve these situations. For example, if an advanced cataract causes a lens to become enlarged, it can push the iris on top of the trabecular meshwork and close it, creating an acute-angle closure.

One potential solution would be to put a tiny hole in the edge of the iris, a peripheral iridotomy, and provide a new exit for fluid. On the other hand, a simple cataract extraction would solve this problem and possibly provide clearer vision as well.

Similarly, glaucoma resulting from a severe inflammatory eye disease, called uveitis, is much improved when the inflammation is brought under control. If the inflammation cannot be controlled, or if anti-inflammatory medications such as steroids increase eye pressure, then tube shunt surgery may be necessary.

If you have uncontrolled diabetic eye disease (called proliferative diabetic retinopathy), your retina can be deprived of oxygen and nutrients. This can lead to a type of secondary glaucoma (called neovascular glaucoma). A large blood clot in the retina or blockage of an artery in the retina can also block the delivery of oxygen and nutrients. In response to the cutoff blood flow, the eye quickly forms new blood vessels. Unfortunately, these new blood vessels tend to be fragile, bleed easily, and grow in an unregulated manner. They can grow over the trabecular meshwork and form a membrane that blocks the eye's normal fluid-filtering apparatus.

This condition can be very difficult to treat. The first goal is to get the abnormal blood vessels to regress. This is done using a laser procedure called pan retinal photocoagulation (PRP), which involves placing up to 2,000 laser spots in the peripheral parts of the retina. Doctors believe this treatment acts by reducing the production of a hormone called vascular endothelial growth factor, which is responsible for the growth of problematic blood vessels.

Laser photocoagulation has many complications, including constriction of the peripheral field of vision and nighttime vision reduction. Recently, medications have been discovered that can block vascular endothelial growth factor when injected into the eye. These medications may reduce neovascular glaucoma, although their effectiveness hasn't been proven yet. If laser retinal treatment does not reduce your eye pressure sufficiently, then tube shunt surgery may help. If, however, your eye has poor vision that is not expected to improve, and you are experiencing discomfort, cyclophotocoagulation may be a better option.

Corneal Transplantation: Complications and Treatments

Before your doctor recommends undergoing a corneal transplant to correct the cloudiness of your cornea, she will evaluate you to determine whether your cornea might be cleared up using another procedure. Corneal clouding of the superficial surface of the cornea sometimes can be corrected using PTK, which is similar to PRK. Potential complications of PTK are much like those of PRK (described in Chapter Four).

The goal of PRK, like LASIK, is to improve the ability of your eye to focus. The primary goal of PTK is not to free you from your need to wear glasses, but to shave away the superficial, cloudy portion of the cornea in order to restore useful vision. Nevertheless, it also may be possible during the same operation to reshape the cornea to improve your ability to focus. This additional corneal adjustment during the PTK procedure may eliminate the need for glasses in appropriate patients.

If PTK or other medical treatments are not options for clearing up your cloudy cornea, you become a potential candidate for a corneal transplant: a delicate procedure in which the central portion of your diseased or damaged cornea is removed and replaced with corneal tissue from a donor.

How Are Corneas Screened for Transplantation?

Corneas used in transplant operations are provided by eye banks. Eye banks get their material from organ donors. Remember the question on the back of your driver's license about organ donation? People who sign this form or otherwise agree to donate their organs help others regain their vision.

The eye bank is responsible for guaranteeing the health of the cornea. It helps assure that the tissue harbors no potentially lethal viruses that can infect the recipient. The donor material is tested for a variety of infectious viruses and agents, including those that cause HIV, hepatitis C, and Creutzfeldt-Jakob disease, the human equivalent of mad cow disease. The eye bank also assures that the donor material is in good shape, that the cornea is clear, and the endothelial cells in its inner segment are healthy.

Too few endothelial cells would lead to corneal clouding in the recipient. Problems with endothelial cells play a central role in an inherited disease called Fuchs' corneal dystrophy, one of the most frequent reasons people need corneal transplants. People with this condition lack a sufficient number of endothelial cells in their cornea to keep it clear.

During a corneal transplant, the central portion of the recipient's cornea is cut out, and the donor cornea is carefully sutured onto the recipient's remaining, peripheral, corneal tissue. The corneal graft needs to be handled carefully and delicately during surgery. Surgical manipulation itself can cause endothelia cell death. The resulting poor-quality tissue can cloud up quickly after the transplant procedure is completed.

Following the operation, your ophthalmologist examines and monitors you for complications. The typical recovery period for a standard cornea transplant can take one to two years and includes use of steroid eyedrops indefinitely.

To prevent infection, antibiotic eyedrops are used for at least a week after your corneal transplant operation. You'll also be using frequent steroid eyedrops. If you have an eyelid condition called blepharitis, you should be treated for it before and after transplant surgery, because this chronic, low-grade infection increases your risk of developing a more serious complication. You may have blepharitis if your eyelids are constantly red, you frequently get morning crusting of the eyelids, and you feel like there is something in your eyes (when there isn't).

If you experience increased cloudy vision, light sensitivity, and discharge from the eye after a corneal transplant, go to your doctor immediately. Your doctor may increase your antibiotic and steroid treatment. Or he may prescribe different antibiotics after testing the antibiotic sensitivity of the bacteria causing the infection. This may be the key to resolving the crisis. Endophthalmitis is also a risk and may require injections of antibiotics directly into the eye.

Suture Complications

The sutures you receive when your new cornea is implanted may remain in your eye for two years and longer. They are removed systematically, over a period of time. On occasion, an inflammation can occur around one or more of the sutures. This is sometimes seen as a spot of redness in the white part of the eye near the problem suture. In this case, the frequency of steroid eyedrops is increased. Adding antibiotics may help, and it may be necessary to remove the troublesome suture before its scheduled removal date. Sometimes one or more of the sutures pokes out, producing a sticky feeling in the eye. Go to your surgeon if you feel this sensation. Although it may feel like it, it is unlikely to be a symptom of a dry eye. The surgeon can remove the suture in a painless office procedure.

Astigmatism

Astigmatism is considered more of a *consequence* of corneal transplant surgery than it is a complication. How difficult it is to correct with glasses depends on the skill of the surgeon. When the surgeon places a suture into the surface of the cornea, it distorts that section of the cornea. This distortion causes light to bend in one particular direction, which is a key feature of astigmatism. Sutures tightened equally and placed directly opposite each other cancel the astigmatism produced by the other. This is where the "art" of corneal surgery is critical.

Very experienced corneal-transplant surgeons minimize astigmatism in patients by choosing the best approach to securing the new cornea and by knowing how many sutures to use and where to secure them. Knowing when, how, and which sutures to remove in the months after surgery also influences the degree of postsurgical astigmatism. Usually your surgeon removes the sutures in a manner that balances the astigmatism. If you have irregular astigmatism, a good surgeon knows which suture to remove and when to remove it to cancel induced irregular astigmatism.

Rejection

Rejection is a real complication of corneal transplantation. It can happen weeks, months, or even years after your surgery. Clouding of vision, redness, eye irritation, and/or pain are all symptoms. If this happens to you, your ophthalmologist will increase the frequency of steroid drops and put you on antirejection eyedrops, such as Restasis (which are also used to treat dry eye). You may also receive the corticosteroid prednisone. If this doesn't work, and your immune system attacks the transplanted cornea, you need another one. Some people have two or three grafts before one is successful.

Glaucoma

Uncontrolled glaucoma poses a high risk for transplant failure. If you have glaucoma and need a corneal transplant, your surgeon must make sure your glaucoma is under complete control before you undergo surgery. Don't be surprised if your ophthalmologist tells you that you need filtration surgery prior to your transplant, even if your pre-existing glaucoma has been under control with glaucoma drops. The filtration surgery is done to assure that your glaucoma is *completely* under control. This minimizes the risks of graft failure and/or worsening glaucoma.

Even after these precautions, it is essential that you faithfully see your ophthalmologist for regular follow-up exams. One among many reasons for this is that the long-term use of steroid eyedrops after corneal transplantation can lead to glaucoma.

Cataracts

Any eye surgery that disrupts the natural environment of the lens can induce cataracts. This is true for corneal transplantation, but the incidence of cataracts after transplant surgery is lower than it is following retinal surgery.

Some patients may need cataract surgery at the same time that their cornea is at risk for failure—Fuchs' corneal dystrophy is the most frequent cause of this situation. If the cataract surgery is performed as an isolated procedure, the cornea will almost surely cloud up afterward, and the patient will need a cornea transplant. If you are one of these patients, your surgeon may strongly suggest you undergo a combined corneal transplant and cataract surgery. This gets you on the way to clear vision more quickly. With the advent of corneal endothelial transplants, you may be able to recover even more quickly.

Corneal Endothelial Transplants: Complications and Solutions

A new technique has been developed that does not require transplantation of the full thickness of the cornea. Corneal endothelial transplantation was developed to treat corneal clouding due to the degeneration of the innermost layer of the cornea, the endothelium. It is only appropriate when the cornea is cloudy due to a problem with the endothelial cell layer in the cornea.

This extremely delicate surgery involves removing the endothelial layer from the recipient and replacing it with donor endothelial tissue. So far, it has been quite successful.

The grafted layer is folded like a taco and inserted through a small incision in the cornea. Once inserted, it is flattened out. A bubble of air is injected to keep the endothelial layer flat against the rest of the cornea until your eye's normal adhesive mechanisms secure it. This novel approach has the advantage of producing little or no astigmatism because no sutures are used. Also, recovery time is significantly faster. But, as with all medical procedures, there are some complications to watch out for.

Endothelial Layer Separation or Folding

The endothelial layer can become separated or detached either during the surgery or a day or two after the procedure. This can happen when the endothelial layer fails to stick because the air bubble evaporates too quickly. It also can occur if the transplanted layer of endothelial tissue slips in the first day or two after surgery, i.e., before the eye's normal adhesive mechanism secures it in place. If this is discovered in the doctor's office, your doctor may inject another sterile air bubble. Or, if necessary, the problem might be fixed with a return to the operating room.

It is critical that there are no folds in the transplanted layer of endothelial cells. It must be absolutely flat to adhere properly and for your sight to be clear upon recovery. If any folds are too large, they disrupt vision. They may also get bigger. If you notice a problem, or if folds are discovered during an exam after surgery, your ophthalmologist may be able to smooth out the endothelial layer using specialized surgical instruments in her office.

Failure

If too few endothelial cells are present in the graft, or if the endothelial cell layer itself is damaged during surgery due to folding and unfolding, then the cornea can become cloudy again. Up to 30 percent of the endothelial cells may die during this type of transplant surgery. Newer, gentler techniques are being investigated, and this complication should be less frequent as these techniques are improved.

Glaucoma

Acute-angle closure glaucoma can be a high risk in the first few days after transplant surgery. This can happen if the air bubble injected to hold down the endothelial cell layer physically interferes with the function of the eye's fluid-filtering apparatus, the trabecular meshwork. This can cause eye pressure to build up quickly. To prevent this from happening, most surgeons perform a PI (described on page 108) during the corneal endothelial transplant surgery.

If you suddenly experience nausea, vomiting, or eye ache as well as develop cloudy or smoky vision and see halos around lights, immediately go to the nearest emergency room with an eye care service if it is after hours, or call your ophthalmologist. If it is acute-angle closure, you need emergency treatment.

Chapter Twelve

Macular Degeneration and Retinal Surgery

The retina is like a motor that powers the visual system. Like an automobile engine, which transforms one type of energy (gasoline) into another (movement), the retina transforms light into electrical energy in the form of nerve impulses. These impulses carry visual information to the brain, where it is processed, integrated, and interpreted.

Macular Degeneration

Several diseases can threaten the retina. At the top of the list is age-related macular degeneration, which is becoming increasingly common as baby boomers age. Encouragingly, there have been great improvements in the past four years in the treatment of one form of this disease called wet macular degeneration. Medication that is injected directly into the vitreous, the gel-like substance filling the back chamber of the eye, is helping many people with this common condition.

Modern medicine offers sight-saving treatments for other retinal problems. Laser surgery, for example, can stop bleeding in the retina, a problem in uncontrolled diabetes when abnormal and fragile blood vessels leak fluid and cause major bleeding episodes.

Sight can also be threatened when membranes and holes grow in the center of the retina, distorting visual images or causing images or letters to "drop out." This damage can be halted by surgical procedures called membrane peel and macular hole repair. Strokes and blood clots in retinal blood vessels that can cause intractable glaucoma and irreversible blindness may be treated with laser and glaucoma surgery. And the prompt, surgical reattachment of a detached retina can prevent irreversible loss of vision.

Treatment of Wet Macular Degeneration

Age-related macular degeneration (ARMD) is the most frequently diagnosed retinal disease among the elderly. By some estimates, 20 percent of people over 75 years of age show signs of it. Its incidence is on the rise as the population ages and we live longer. Macular degeneration is caused by the accumulation of large lipid deposits that interfere with the delivery of nutrients to cells in the central part of the retina. These deposits cause the cells to degenerate.

The wet form of macular degeneration can result in a relatively rapid and sometimes devastating loss of central vision. It may cause a blur to appear where you should see someone's face, or you may find that entire words or letters disappear from a page you are reading. This form of the disease is thought to occur because abnormal blood vessels develop in the damaged retina. These easily bleeding vessels leak fluid or blood and cause massive disruption to the cellular architecture of the macula, leading to the sudden loss of central vision. A diagnosis of wet macular degeneration before 2004 was almost certain to be followed by a devastating loss of vision.

Laser Treatments

The first attempt to treat the wet form of macular degeneration used destructive laser energy to destroy, or burn away, abnormal blood vessels. The results of large, multiple clinical trials indicated that if patients with certain types of wet macular degeneration received this treatment, their vision's deterioration would slow down or even stop. However, while this worked for quite a number of patients, the complications were great and sometimes outweighed the benefits of the treatment.

Unfortunately, this early destructive laser therapy did not improve anyone's vision. Instead, the laser burn treatment itself left remaining vision even worse. Nevertheless, the treatment did succeed in stabilizing the remaining vision for five years or so, compared to people who didn't receive the treatment. People with wet macular degeneration were left with a choice. They could either experience progressively poor vision over the course of a few years or experience a sudden loss of vision but with less degradation during the next five years.

Laser treatment was also used in cases when wet macular degeneration did not affect the center of the visual field. This treatment left a permanent blind spot in the periphery of the visual field. Another complication, in addition to the side effect of vision loss at the site of the laser burn, was increased recurrence of the abnormal blood vessels and further bleeding. Moreover, this type of laser therapy was not effective in all types of wet macular degeneration. Despite these drawbacks, laser therapy may still have a role in the treatment of certain types of wet macular degeneration and related eye disorders that do not affect central vision.

Light Therapy

The FDA approved another treatment for certain types of wet ARMD in 2003, and it is still used in some cases today. Photodynamic therapy (PDT) begins with the intravenous injection of a blood-vessel-staining dye into the patient. The dye accumulates in the abnormal blood vessels that form in wet ARMD. Laser light is then directed at the stained blood vessels within a few minutes of the injection. The laser light activates the dye, marking the abnormal blood vessels in the area of the macular degeneration. Once activated, the dye destroys the leaky vessels. An advantage of this approach is its specificity; it does not destroy healthy tissue surrounding the damaged blood vessels. Studies involving many patients revealed that this treatment was superior to standard laser therapy in stabilizing the vision loss in wet ARMD. However, PDT carries a risk of sudden vision loss as a result of laser burns (1 to 4 percent). While it is not effective for all types of wet ARMD, it does work when certain architectural features form in the retina. The results of PDT are temporary, and the procedure may have to be repeated every three months or so.

The most frequent complication of PDT is related to the dye used in the procedure. It leaves the skin excessively sensitive to light and subject to severe sunburn. If you have this procedure, you should not expose your eyes, face, or skin to the sun for a week after treatment. Some patients (for no clear reason) have experienced lower backaches after the treatment. Complications associated with the intravenous site itself include pain and bruising. Applying ice to the injection site is usually enough to handle these complaints.

Injection Therapy

When tissue lacks nutrients, the body responds by releasing specific hormones to make sure the deprived tissue gets what it needs. One of the most important of these hormones is a protein called vascular endothelial growth factor (VEGF). This hormone stimulates the formation and growth of new blood vessels. Degenerating cells in the retina send out chemical signals that tell the body they are not getting enough nutrients. The body responds by sending VEGF to the area to stimulate the formation of blood vessels. Unfortunately, in cases of ARMD, the blood vessels that form in response to VEGF are not organized and are very fragile. This means they grow in an unorganized fashion and bleed easily.

To treat this condition, pharmaceutical companies began looking for molecules that inhibit the action of VEGF. So far, all of the compounds they have found have to be injected directly into the back segment (vitreous) of the eye. The first compound to be developed is called Macugen (pegaptanib) and is marketed by Pfizer Pharmaceuticals. Macugen acts by preventing VEGF from attaching to its "docking site" or receptor. If it can't link up to the site of blood vessel formation, VEGF can't form new blood vessels.

The results of large clinical trials indicate that Macugen slows the progression of visual loss in a large majority of patients with wet ARMD better than laser or light therapy does. Moreover, about 6 out of 100 patients had modest improvement in their vision. This finding was very exciting, because it was the first time anyone had seen improvement in this disease. In general, however, patients continued to experience deterioration of vision, albeit less than untreated patients did.

Newer VEGF inhibitors are now available. The Genentech compound Lucentis (generic name ranibizumab) was approved by the FDA in 2006 for treating ARMD. The clinical results of several studies have been very exciting so far. First, the treatment allowed almost 90 percent of the patients tested to either maintain or even improve their vision compared to 60 percent of patients whose vision was maintained by PDT. The most encouraging result is that a large minority of patients, up to 40 percent, actually experienced improved vision after injection of Lucentis.

More good news is that most, if not all, types of wet ARMD may respond to treatment with VEGF inhibitor compounds. Researchers are working now to determine how often and for how long injections should be given. For example, should people be treated monthly for the rest of their lives, or should they be treated monthly for three or six months, and then wait until the abnormality returns?

While these treatments have produced very exciting results, they are not a panacea, since only a minority—albeit a large one—experiences improved vision. Unfortunately, some patients do not respond to the treatment, and their vision continues to deteriorate.

Some ophthalmologists are using a compound closely related to Lucentis, called Avastin. This medicine has been approved for the treatment of early colon cancer, but not for ARMD. It works in the same way Lucentis does, but it has the advantage of being much cheaper ($150 versus $2,000 per injection). Since some insurance companies claim Lucentis is experimental and won't pay for its use, some ophthalmologists have been using Avastin on an off-label basis to treat their patients.

Complications of such treatments are typically related to the injection site, where pain and bleeding have occurred in some patients. The procedure is done under sterile conditions, and antibiotic eyedrops are given for a few days after surgery. Retinal bleeding and retinal tears are rare complications that usually resolve by themselves. If necessary, a retinal tear can be repaired by laser treatment to prevent it from becoming a detachment. Endophthalmitis, a very serious and potentially blinding inflammatory infection, is also rare, occurring only in about 1 in 4,500 cases.

Avastin, when injected intravenously in people who have colon cancer, increases the risk of embolic (arteriosclerotic) strokes. Theoretically, injections of the compound into the eye could lead to trace levels of the drug in the general circulatory system. In large clinical trials conducted with Lucentis, there was a two- to fourfold increased incidence of stroke in patients taking the higher dose, but the overall risk was small: about 1 or 2 out of 100 patients. People who have had previous strokes are probably more at risk. Most ophthalmologists discuss these risks before treatment. Obviously, since most of the patients who have wet ARMD are elderly, this is an important point of discussion.

Dry versus Wet Macular Degeneration

Nearly all cases of macular degeneration start out as the dry form of the disease, and 85 percent of them remain dry. It is caused by shrinkage of a layer of the retina called the retinal pigment epithelium. In the early stage, it does not affect vision. In the intermediate stage, you may find yourself needing more light for some tasks such as reading. In the advanced stage, you see a blurry spot in the center of your visual field, which gets bigger and more opaque as the disease progresses.

Dry macular degeneration can turn into the wet form of the disease suddenly and without warning. About 15 percent of people with the dry form go on to develop the wet form. "Wet" refers to the presence of fluid leaking out of abnormal, fragile blood vessels, which form under the central part of the retina or the macula, which provides your central, as opposed to peripheral, vision. The wet form causes the most serious loss of vision in age-related macular degeneration.

Treatment of Dry Macular Degeneration

At first, vision may be affected only minimally in the dry form of macular degeneration, but it can slowly progress over months or years. It can cause letters to appear distorted and straight lines to appear curvy. There is, unfortunately, no approved, effective treatment for the nonexudative dry form of macular degeneration. Attempts at laser and other therapies have been either ineffective or have made vision worse. But because the progression of the disease is often quite slow, patients can learn to adapt to the changes by using their peripheral vision. And there is a preventive treatment that may reduce progressive visual loss by about 20 percent: daily use of a specific formulation of vitamins and micronutrients called the Age-Related Eye Disease Study (AREDS) formula.

Vitamin Therapy
The best option available for preventing or slowing the progression of dry macular degeneration is a combination of vitamins and micronutrients. A large clinical trial involving almost 5,000 patients evaluated whether a combination of high-dose vitamins and micronutrients containing specific concentrations of vitamin E, beta-carotene, vitamin C, zinc, and cobalt protected patients from ARMD.

The AREDS evaluated patients who had an average of six years of treatment over the course of a decade. It concluded that the supplements reduced the risk of disease progression by 25 percent in people with an intermediate form of ARMD in both eyes or advanced ARMD in one eye. It also reduced by 20 percent their chances of losing more of their vision. It isn't known if people who have mild or no ARMD would benefit from the AREDS vitamins.

Should You Use Supplements to Prevent Age-Related Macular Degeneration?

AREDS vitamins are available in the vitamin or eye sections of pharmacies. Smokers should consider taking a formula without beta-carotene, since this compound increases the risk of lung cancer in people who smoke. Before taking these and other supplements, talk to your ophthalmologist and family doctor. They consider the benefits and potential complicating factors based on your medical history and other medications you are taking.

A new clinical trial, AREDS II, will test more specific nutrients and different doses. Many other micronutrients have been suggested as treatments for ARMD. The challenge of conducting good clinical trials that test each of them and determine which concentration would be most effective would, unfortunately, run into the billions of dollars.

Diabetic Retinopathy: Complications and Solutions

Uncontrolled diabetes can result in a myriad of health problems: Damaged peripheral nerves can lead to toe and leg sores that don't heal and eventually require amputation, kidney failure requires dialysis, and retinal bleeding and swelling can threaten sight. Diabetes can affect the eye, because failure to regulate glucose in the blood, a consequence of uncontrolled diabetes, causes blood vessels in the retina to leak.

Leakage into the central part of the retina, the macula, causes the cells there to swell. This condition is called macular edema. Leaking blood vessels starve the retina of oxygen and nutrients, which is a condition called ischemia. As described earlier in this chapter, ischemia stimulates the formation of vascular endothelial growth factor (VEGF) , which in turn stimulates the formation of abnormal blood vessels. Fragile and prone to bleeding, these vessels can cause a vitreous hemorrhage, which can blur vision completely. Vision suffers if swelling is prolonged. If this happens, your ophthalmologist is able to see spot hemorrhages, lipid (fat) deposits, and swelling in your retina. This stage of the disease is called nonproliferative diabetic retinopathy (NPDR) because no new blood vessels are forming. Proliferative diabetic retinopathy (PDR) is a more advanced condition and carries an increased risk of blindness due to the continuing formation of new, unstable blood vessels.

Swelling of the Retina

Prevention is the key in diabetic retinopathy. This is achieved by closely monitoring and controlling glucose levels in the blood. In NPDR, treatment is aimed at macular edema if present. Multiple clinical studies have shown that an office procedure involving light and painless laser treatment (focal laser) to the area of leaking blood vessels prevents further leakage, dries up the macula, and stabilizes and sometimes improves vision that is affected by the macular edema. Some patients may need multiple laser treatments to stop the leakage.

Complications from this type of laser treatment may include a permanent central blind spot if the laser is aimed incorrectly or if the patient moves during treatment. Worsening vision is another complication, especially after multiple laser treatments, which may leave some retinal scarring. There are no treatments for these complications, but with both eyes open the brain learns to ignore the blind spot or scotoma.

If the macular edema cannot be controlled by laser treatment, injection of a steroid into the superficial layers of the retina to reduce inflammation sometimes helps. This type of injection can cause an increase in eye pressure, which, in turn, can cause glaucoma, cataracts, and sometimes upper eyelid droop. Glaucoma can be treated with eyedrops (Chapter Eleven), cataracts with surgery (Chapters Seven and Eight), and the eyelid droop (Chapter Nine) with an eyelid lift, if necessary.

If the laser or laser and steroid combination does not work, you may have as an option a type of surgery called vitrectomy, in which the gel-like material in the back part of the eye, the vitreous, is removed and replaced with a physiologically balanced fluid. Complications of a vitrectomy include a likely cataract (Chapters Seven and Eight), a low risk of a retinal detachment (Chapter Eight), and a very low risk of an infection called endophthalmitis (Chapter Eight).

Retinal Bleeding

PDR (proliferative diabetic retinopathy) is a very serious condition and, depending on its stage, can carry a high risk of blindness due to the presence of unstable, abnormal blood vessels. These leaky blood vessels can cause severe loss of vision as blood from the vitreous hemorrhage enters the back chamber of the eye.

Initial treatment calls for waiting for the blood to be absorbed, followed by extensive application of laser burns to the edges of the retina. This procedure, called PRP, causes the unwanted blood vessels to disappear or regress, perhaps by inhibiting VEGF. Usually 1,200 to 2,000 laser spots are applied either in one application or in multiple, sequential sessions. If you have macular edema along with PDR, then the macular edema needs to be treated with a focal laser before the doctor attempts photocoagulation, otherwise the swelling will get worse. Applying photocoagulation over several sessions may also decrease the symptoms of night-vision problems and peripheral field defects.

Most patients are able to tolerate the treatment using numbing eyedrops, although sometimes a numbing injection is required to control pain. Acetaminophen (such as Tylenol) usually will take care of any residual pain after the laser treatment.

Potential problems following PRP include loss of peripheral vision and decreased night vision, both of which are the result of laser burns that destroy the retina around its edges. This may, in turn, cause a mild loss of vision as well. If glare turns out to be a complication, use of antireflective coating on glasses may help counter it.

Not treating PDR can lead to retinal detachment, which requires one or multiple retinal detachment surgeries. This happens because the abnormal blood vessels form sticky membranes that pull on the retina and create what is called a tractional detachment. Tractional retinal detachments are difficult to treat. Another potential consequence of PDR is a form of glaucoma called neovascular glaucoma, in which an abnormal blood vessel membrane forms over, and closes off, the filtering mechanism of the eye. PRP is the treatment of choice here as well. Neovascular glaucoma is not easy to treat, and prognosis can be poor.

A Promising New Treatment for PDR and Neovascular Glaucoma?

There have been several successful attempts at using the injection of VEGF-inhibiting compounds to treat PDR and neovascular glaucoma. These new medications are sometimes used in combination with laser treatment. Although there have been no clinical studies to compare Lucentis or similar medications against PRP in PDR, the use of VEGF inhibitors may potentially cause fewer complications since they do not appear to be destructive to the retina. Instead, these injected compounds target the growth factor that induces blood vessel formation. Their disadvantage is that the injections may need to be repeated for a long time.

If vitreous bleeding is persistent and fails to clear up, or if it recurs despite proper PRP treatment, then surgical removal of the gel in the back chamber of the eye, a vitrectomy, is the next option for treatment. This is often followed by intraoperative PRP laser treatment.

Treatment of Macular Holes and Epiretinal Membranes

Some problems can occur between the vitreous gel, which is normally attached to the retina, and the retina itself. Most of these are attributed to aging, but some occur for unknown reasons. The vitreous is normally attached to the retina at several points, including the macula in the center, the blood vessels, the optic nerve, and the periphery. A sudden separation of the vitreous from the retina causes you to see floaters that are sometimes preceded by light flashes. This is very common and most often happens because the vitreous gel liquefies at its center and degenerates. As the eye moves in its socket, the liquid part of the vitreous sloshes back and forth. This causes the vitreous to tug on its remaining attachments to the retina. Further separation in the periphery can pull a piece of peripheral retina away from its secured position and cause a retinal tear, which can become a detachment. Retinal detachment is described later in this chapter.

A slower separation of the vitreous from the macula may cause your central vision to blur or letters in a word you are reading to disappear. This is the result of something called a macular hole. If some vitreous cells are left behind after the vitreous separates from the retina, they can grow between the vitreous and the macula. There they can form a membrane over the macula that distorts the macula itself. This is known as an epiretinal membrane. Symptoms include image distortion with bowing or curving of letters, doubling of images in the affected eye, and something called micropsia, in which letters in the center of a word appear smaller than those on either side. Surgery is usually not used to treat epiretinal membrane or macular hole unless vision is worse than 20/50 or you cannot tolerate the distortion of your vision.

Gas Injections

Outpatient surgery for macular holes is usually done by first removing the vitreous gel and then injecting sterile gas to create a bubble that blocks the hole. The success rate for this procedure is very high: up to 90 percent of patients see improvement. The timing of the surgery is critical; visual recovery is much better in cases of recently formed holes than when holes are older than six months or so. You must lie facedown most of the time for the first week or so following the procedure to make sure the gas bubble presses against the macula.

It is not fun to lie in this position for such a long time, and *all* patients hate doing it—but it is required. Otherwise, the hole will remain open. There are break periods, but the longer you stay in the correct position, the more successful your surgery is likely to be.

Your surgeon may be able to supply you with a pillow that has an opening in the center into which you can place your nose and face to make your recovery more comfortable. If you can't get one from your doctor, you can try to arrange a couple of neck pillows, like those used when sleeping on airplanes, to create a donut shape, which supports your head while you lie facedown.

Complications of macular hole surgery include cataracts necessitating cataract surgery, reopening of the macular hole, which would require another surgery to close it, retinal tear and detachment, which can be treated with laser or sclera buckle surgery, and secondary glaucoma, which can be treated with eyedrops.

Vitreous Surgery

Vitrectomy is the most commonly performed retinal surgery. An outpatient procedure, it is performed with local or general anesthesia. Probes are inserted into the posterior segment of the eye. These are used to microcut the vitreous gel and to suction gel pieces out of the eye. The vitreous then is replaced with a buffered salt solution.

Vitrectomy is used to remove blood clots or hemorrhages in people with diabetes and to clear bacteria and pus in cases of endophthalmitis. It also is the preliminary step in other retinal surgeries, such as the closure of a macular hole or the removal of an epiretinal membrane, as described earlier in this chapter.

As mentioned previously, the most common complication of vitrectomy is formation or worsening of a cataract. In fact, up to 90 percent of patients develop a significant cataract within two years of their vitrectomy surgery. The solution is cataract surgery, which typically carries no additional risk of complications over normal cataract surgery. Vitrectomy also is associated with a 20-percent risk of developing glaucoma. Be sure to watch for signs of retinal tears and detachment (see Chapter Eight and a later section in this chapter). There is less chance of developing the infection called endophthalmitis following a vitrectomy than there is following cataract or glaucoma surgery.

Treatment of Blood Clots and Strokes

A blood clot in a vein is not an uncommon occurrence in the eye. Uncontrolled high blood pressure raises the risks considerably. Both small and large veins can become blocked.

Blockages in small veins can decrease vision and cause problems with your peripheral vision, but these defects can improve with time and, if necessary, with laser treatment.

Large veins experience two types of blockages. The first, called an ischemic central retinal vein occlusion (CRVO), is painless but causes permanent vision loss and leads to secondary glaucoma and retinal bleeding. The second, called nonischemic CRVO, is less devastating and offers a good chance of improvement.

Laser Treatments

A blood clot in a small vein can cause inflammatory swelling in the retina, which blurs vision. This typically occurs soon after the clot forms but recedes two to three months afterward. If the blurring and the swelling persist, light laser treatment can decrease the swelling. Risk from this laser treatment is minimal unless the treatment is too strong or the blood clot inadvertently falls onto the central part of the retina or the macula. This can produce a blind spot called a scotoma.

A blood clot in a large vein produces a high risk of developing glaucoma due to the formation of abnormal vessels on the fluid-filtering mechanism of the eye, the trabecular meshwork. These unwanted blood vessels can be destroyed with PRP, the same scatter laser treatment described in the previous section on retinal bleeding. Since neovascular glaucoma does not respond readily to eyedrops or simple filtration surgery, it is best addressed early with PRP as soon as these abnormal blood vessels are recognized and before eye pressure goes up.

Blocked Arteries

Arteries, like veins, in the retina can become blocked. If a small or branch retinal artery is blocked, vision in the peripheral field corresponding to the area of the occlusion is affected. Unfortunately, there is no treatment or recovery when this happens. If the larger, central retinal artery is blocked, it causes a devastating, sudden, painless loss of vision: sometimes from 20/20 to barely being able to perceive light. Again, with no textbook remedies for this problem, your ophthalmologist should observe you closely for any signs of developing neovascular glaucoma.

Some ophthalmologists have tried an experimental procedure to treat this sight-threatening event. They have injected a clot-busting drug called t-PA into the retinal artery to restore blood flow. This must be done within two hours or so of the onset of the attack. And some studies indicate that reducing the eye pressure drastically within one hour of a central retinal artery blockage can improve visual outcome by permitting the cholesterol plaque to flow to smaller arteries with less devastating consequence to vision. This treatment, it must be stressed, is not standard procedure.

If you have experienced a blocked artery in your eye, you should have a full cardiovascular and brain workup to make sure you don't have more threatening cholesterol plaques in your neck arteries or in your heart that could potentially cause a stroke or heart attack.

Injections Following Blocked Blood Vessels

Ophthalmologists have tried injecting VEGF inhibitors, such as Lucentis, into the vitreous to prevent the development of neovascular glaucoma in patients with the ischemic form of large retinal vein blockages. Recent studies, however, indicate that Lucentis is no more effective than scatter laser treatment, and the results may not last as long, creating the need for repeated injections.

Patients who develop macular edema after vein blockage, and who do not respond to laser treatment, may improve dramatically with steroid injection into the vitreous cavity. So far, however, no large clinical trial data are available to document this effect. Of course, the potential complications of steroid injections, both glaucoma and cataract, have to be weighed against the possible benefits.

Treatment of Retinal Tears and Retinal Detachments

Rarely, when the vitreous gel separates or detaches from its normal point of attachment to the retina, it can pull a piece of retina out with it, causing a retinal tear. You may notice light flashes and/or a floater that looks like a string, bug, spider web, or a running black spot. If you see anything like this, visit an ophthalmologist immediately.

The tear itself might be inconsequential if it happens in the periphery of the retina. It does, however, increase the risk of a retinal detachment. This happens when the fluid core of the vitreous gel seeps behind the retinal tear and slowly separates the retina from its normal attachment to the back of the eyeball. This deprives the retina of nutrition, causing it to atrophy, which leads to permanent loss of vision.

One symptom of a retinal detachment, in addition to floaters and light flashes, is a sense that a curtain or veil has fallen over your visual field. The veil can cover the side of your visual field or—more ominously—the center, when the macula itself is detached. This is a true eye emergency, and surgical repair is necessary. If you don't get medical attention within three days of the occurrence of a macular-involving retinal detachment, you will have a poor chance of recovering.

Lasers

Peripheral retinal tears are treated with laser burns, which essentially "spot-weld" the retina with scar tissue that holds it in place. A blind spot may develop if the area of the tear is not in the far periphery. While this procedure decreases the risk of detachment, it doesn't guarantee that it won't happen again. Be sure to see your ophthalmologist for regular, dilated, retinal exams.

Gas, Belts, and Buckles

Surgery is required when fluid seeps behind a detached retina. If the detachment is small and shallow enough, it is sometimes possible to push it back into place so it can reattach itself. This office procedure involves injecting a sterile gas bubble into the eye and holding your head in such a way that the bubble presses against the retina.

Larger or deeper detachments require outpatient surgery conducted under either local or general anesthesia. This procedure involves the injection of a gas bubble and the insertion of encircling bands, called scleral buckles, that act like belts to squeeze the outer part of the eye and the retina together. At the same time, the gas bubble pushes on the retina from the inside. To attach the encircling bands, the surgeon must detach the muscles that control eye movement. She then inserts the bands in pockets created in the part of the eyeball exposed by detaching the muscles. The bands are then tightened and the eye muscles reattached.

Postoperative complications of scleral buckle surgery include pain, sometimes requiring narcotic analgesics and, most commonly, increased nearsightedness. The nearsightedness occurs because the length of the eye increases as the scleral buckles squeeze it. As a result, your eyeglass prescription must be adjusted. Other potential complications include worsening cataracts, additional retinal detachments, glaucoma, upper eyelid droop, and double vision with strabismus. Sometimes strabismus surgery (Chapter Ten) is needed to properly align the eye and correct its imaging ability.

There is a small chance that the scleral buckles could erode, in which case they may need to be replaced. An infection called orbital cellulitis is also a possibility with scleral buckle surgery, and if this occurs, it is treated by topical and oral antibiotics.

Chapter Thirteen

How to Find and Choose the Right Doctor

For much of the last century, physicians enjoyed an especially elevated status in society. In many cases doctors told patients only what they thought their patients should know about the nature and seriousness of their illnesses. Patients were inclined not to question their doctors. Today, however, patients are more likely to act as medical consumers than children. This improved relationship places a responsibility on patients, the responsibility to locate and evaluate their health care providers.

What You Should Know about Your Doctor

The selection of the person to operate on or otherwise treat your eyes should not be left to random choice. There are five factors to consider when you decide who should perform your surgery or provide additional treatment, if required:

1. Educational and professional credentials
2. Skill and experience in performing the procedure or providing treatment
3. Evidence of willingness to work with you after the surgery, if necessary
4. Past and pending disciplinary history
5. Personal compatibility

You may need to consult a second doctor after your operation if your condition does not respond to treatment provided by your original surgeon and/or if your surgeon is not responsive to your needs.

Educational and Professional Credentials

Some basic facts you should know about a professional eye care provider are what type of degree or degrees he has earned and where and when he earned them. Newly trained surgeons can offer the latest in surgical care while experienced surgeons who keep up with advances in their field appeal to many patients. You may also want to know what type of internship, residency, fellowship, or other training he has had. It is reassuring to know about the physician's certification to practice, which includes medical licensing information and proof of board certification. Sources of this information are described later in this chapter.

The three main types of eye care professionals are ophthalmologists, optometrists, and opticians. An ophthalmologist is a Doctor of Medicine (MD) or Doctor of Osteopathy (DO). As a licensed physician, an ophthalmologist can diagnose and treat eye diseases, perform surgery, give eye examinations, and write prescriptions for medications as well as corrective lenses.

Ophthalmologists are licensed by state licensing boards. A state licensing board can confirm for you an individual physician's credentials.

Your surgeon should also be board-certified or, if recently graduated, at least board-eligible. This means she has undergone additional training, passed or is eligible to take an examination that tests her knowledge in a specialized field of medicine, and takes part in continuing education programs to maintain expertise that goes beyond the practice of basic medicine. The American Board of Ophthalmology, through the American Board of Medical Specialties, confers board certification to ophthalmologists.

An optometrist has earned a doctorate in Optometry (OD) in a four-year postgraduate program. He can perform eye exams, write prescriptions for eyeglasses and contact lenses, diagnose eye diseases, and in some states prescribe medications for some of those diseases. She also can provide pre- and postsurgical care and, in a few states, perform certain eye surgeries. Many optometrists sell glasses, contact lenses, and frames as well.

Good optometrists are highly skilled and aware of the most recent advances in contact lenses and spectacle correction. Skilled optometrists are also excellent diagnosticians of common eye diseases.

Unlike an ophthalmologist, an optometrist cannot practice general medicine. Ophthalmologists are physicians and surgeons first and have to go to medical school and go through additional training through residency before they become independent. Optometrists do not go to medical school and are therefore not physicians.

It is important to recognize, however, that the decision to license an optometrist to prescribe certain medications or perform some types of surgery is essentially a political rather than a medical one. All that is needed is for a state government to grant permission. For example, optometrists are licensed to perform certain eye surgeries in Oklahoma. Optometrists practicing in Oklahoma, however, are not trained differently from optometrists practicing in states that do not give them permission to operate except for taking courses or apprenticing with an opthalmologist in the surgical procedure. Qualified optometrists are usually certified by the American Board of Optometry.

You might also encounter an eye care professional who is a Certified Ophthalmic Technician (COT). These technicians may be highly skilled and assist ophthalmologists and optometrists in caring for patients by testing eye pressure and vision and performing many important ancillary tests.

Opticians typically dispense and make eyeglasses. They take prescriptions written by ophthalmologists and optometrists and manufacture the lenses, add various coatings, and sell the glasses. A skilled optician knows how to fit glasses so your visual angle is perfectly aligned with the center of the lenses.

They can learn their trade by taking college or university classes, earning an associate's degree from a two-year college, or receiving apprenticeship training. Some states license opticians. The American Board of Opticianry and the National Contact Lens Examiners offer certification exams for opticians.

Skill and Experience

Make sure your doctor has the expertise and skills to give you the best treatment you can find and afford. Board certification is one indication that she is qualified. Reputation among patients and other eye care professionals is another. Consider the number of procedures the doctor has performed and how long he has been practicing. While this is important, remember that newly trained surgeons often have had more exposure to cutting-edge procedures than older surgeons have. This is why it is important for all doctors to continue their education and training at all stages of their careers.

Ascertain how often she treats symptoms like yours and how many times she has performed the operation.

Other factors to consider are any teaching experience or academic appointments, hospital affiliations, and scholarly journal publications as well as continuing education and training the doctor may have. Academic appointments, of course, aren't crucial. Some academic ophthalmologists have actually performed fewer surgeries than their colleagues practicing in the community. Often, surgery in an academic center is performed by an ophthalmologist-in-training, a resident, or a fellow, who is supervised by a more senior surgeon. In addition to practicing medicine, academic ophthalmologists are often involved in basic research or laboratory studies of various eye diseases and are therefore called on to speak at various seminars. You also might want to consider any special citations, awards, recognition by colleagues, and membership in professional organizations, advocacy groups or community organizations.

Willingness to Work with You after the Surgery

This is a critical issue. Find out if the surgeon limits his contribution to surgery itself, while delegating all before-surgery and after-surgery care to others, such as optometrists. This is called co-management. If so, will you only see the surgeon when referred back by the optometrist? Ask about comanagement. Does the optometrist benefit financially by referring you to the surgeon and seeing you after surgery? Does the optometrist benefit financially for not having to refer you back to the surgeon for after-care? Is the surgeon so busy that he doesn't have the time or inclination to see you? While comanagement itself is not harmful, it is the attitude that a caring doctor can offer you that is important in this situation.

Ask the doctor and members of his staff what their policy is regarding enhancement surgery and treatment of postsurgical complications, if they occur. Will they be satisfied, for example, if your vision is 20/20 after LASIK surgery, but you are bothered by glare or poor night vision a year after surgery? Ask how they would treat such a condition.

Personal Compatibility

Before, during, and after surgery or other treatment, you need to feel comfortable and relaxed enough around the doctor and her staff to ask questions and reduce the anxiety that can accompany a visit to the doctor. This means you have to have at least a basic level of rapport with the doctor and the office personnel. If the doctor or someone else you have to work with closely makes you so uncomfortable and adds to the stress of your treatment, you should weigh this factor carefully when making your selection. This applies when choosing a surgeon to perform your initial surgery as well as when selecting a doctor you might need to consult if you have postsurgical complications.

Of course, doctors should not be expected to coddle patients, but they should be able to make them comfortable, answer questions, and reassure them before and immediately after a treatment. Other staff members should be available to answer routine questions and provide help in a friendly manner. The helpfulness, friendliness, organization and competence of the office staff is a reflection of the doctor in charge and serves as an indication of the importance the practice places on patient care. If you feel comfortable with the doctor and the people in the doctor's office, you have satisfied an important requirement for finding a source of good medical care. If you don't feel comfortable, consult another physician.

Disciplinary History

If a physician has a record of disciplinary action, it means a medical organization, a state medical agency, or a federal regulatory agency has determined that she has violated one or more of their rules or regulations. The doctor, for example, might have broken the law or violated rules of professional and moral conduct. If you suspect this might mean that the physician has a personal flaw that could interfere with his ability to provide the best treatment for you, you can either find out more about the alleged or actual violation by asking the physician about it or seek treatment from another doctor.

If a background check turns up indications of criminal activity or convictions, malpractice judgments, past or pending board suspensions or disciplinary actions, consider how these findings could affect the medical care you hope to receive. Sometimes patients who do not have legitimate claims sue a doctor, and such suits should not reflect unfairly on the physician's reputation. But if an individual has been sued multiple times, you should find out why.

Questions You Should Ask When Deciding on a Doctor

The questions you ask before deciding on a doctor depend on the information you need to gather about the doctor's background, the procedure you will undergo, and your medical history. It's a good idea whenever you consult a doctor or other professional to write down all of your concerns and questions before you visit the office. This helps you avoid getting sidetracked or forgetting something you wanted to ask before you leave.

Your questions should be related to four of the five topics outlined earlier: educational and professional credentials, skill and experience performing the procedure you need, evidence of willingness to work with you after the surgery if necessary, and past and pending disciplinary history. Your questions concerning the fifth topic, personal compatibility, are answered by the impression you get while talking to the doctor and others in the office.

Below are some sample questions to ask if you are considering surgery or looking for a doctor to treat an ophthalmologic condition. If you do a little research using the resources and Web sites listed later in this chapter, you won't need to ask the doctor all of these questions directly, although you certainly can if you prefer or need to. Be sure, however, to ask any questions that directly relate to the treatment you might receive and to your case in particular.

Educational and Professional Credentials

Where and when did you get your training? How do you keep up with new developments and techniques? To what professional organizations do you belong? What is your board certification?

Skill, Experience and Ability to Perform the Procedure You Need

When did you start performing surgery or treating cases like mine? How many procedures have you done? What is your complication rate? What is your success rate? What type of complications have you encountered and how have you treated them? Have any of your patients developed eye infections following treatment? Was the source of infection identified and eliminated? Are you familiar with and able to perform different types of refractive eye surgeries so that you can recommend the best option for me?

A doctor who says that he has never had complications is either lying or has done too few surgeries. Complications come with the job. In fact, complications are statistically linked to experience. The more operations a surgeon has done, the higher the complication rate. For example, cataract surgery carries a complication rate of 1 in 100 for a retinal detachment. A surgeon who has done 100 cataract surgeries has had fewer retinal detachments than one who has performed 10,000 cataract surgeries.

Obviously, a surgeon should not have a complication rate at variance with the number of procedures he has performed. A surgeon with

100 cataract surgeries and 10 retinal detachments (instead of the statistically expected one retinal detachment) should have a pretty good explanation for the discrepancy.

Evidence of Willingness to Work with You after Your Surgery

Will you continue to treat me if I am not satisfied with the results of my surgery? How long after surgery will I be able to bring a complication to your notice for treatment? How much will treatment for complications, if any, cost me? Does enhancement or touch-up surgery cost extra? How long after the first surgery will I be eligible for enhancement surgery at a reduced rate, if you charge extra for it? Do you break down individual expenses on your bills, or is everything lumped together?

Remember, any experienced surgeon has had difficult cases that resulted in complications. The key is how the doctor handled the complications. Repeated poor outcomes are a cause for concern.

Past and Pending Disciplinary History

You can ask a doctor if she has had any disciplinary actions taken against her in the past or if there are any that are pending. This might seem like a rude question to some people, but it isn't as long as you ask it in a respectful, nonaccusatory tone. You have the right to know. If a doctor takes offense, it is a good indication you should move on to the next one on the list of those you are considering. Also, you don't need to ask the doctor all of the above questions; members of the doctor's staff can answer some of them, and you can gather other information from state medical boards and other resources listed later in this chapter.

Resources to Help You Find the Right Doctor

Some complications of eye surgery can be corrected by an enhancement procedure or other medical treatment, such as eyedrops. Between 5 and 15 percent of LASIK surgeries, for example, might require a touch-up surgical session according to the American Academy of Opthalmology. Often the surgeon who performed the original procedure can correct the problem. In some difficult-to-treat complications, however, the person who performed the original procedure may not be able to correct the problem with additional surgery or other medical treatment. If this is true in your case, ask your physician to recommend another doctor who has experience treating complications such as yours.

You can expand your search by asking other eye care professionals you have worked with in the past, including your family doctor, optometrist, or ophthalmologist, whom they would recommend. The candidates should have experience performing refractive or other surgery, or if you have already had surgery, treating postsurgical complications. Ask these other eye care professionals which of their colleagues have excellent reputations.

Also ask friends, family, and acquaintances if they know of anyone who has had a successful surgery or been successfully treated and found a doctor they liked. If you have no luck there—or even if you do but want a larger pool of potential doctors to choose from—begin searching online or at your local library. Visit the Web sites of the medical practices you find, if they have any, and read what they have to offer. Then call them and ask questions on the phone and/or schedule a consultation after you have done some basic research into the doctor's background. Remember that a name turned up by referral or by research is still only a candidate for you until you have determined that the doctor is experienced and qualified to help you.

Other potentially useful sources of candidates for your consideration are the Web sites of The American Society of Cataract and Refractive Surgery (ASCRS) and the American Academy of Ophthalmology (AAO). Both can provide the names of potential candidates for you to evaluate. Be sure to specify "refractive surgery" under "specialty" if you are thinking about LASIK or other cosmetic eye surgery.

When you find the names and contact information of doctors on these sites, ask them if they have experience treating your symptoms or performing the surgery you want. You can find doctors all over the country by entering zip codes of regions you are willing to travel to and by describing the medical specialty that most closely matches your needs. The AAO site is "Find an Eye MD" (www.aao.org/find_eyemd.cfm) and the ASCRS site is "Find a Surgeon" (www.ascrs.org/Find-A-Surgeon.cfm). Both offer information based on name, location, or specialty. The AAO's options for searching by specialty include cataract, cornea and external diseases, conjunctivitis/eyelids, contact lenses, glaucoma, comprehensive ophthalmology, low-vision rehabilitation, medical retina, or neuro-ophthalmology. The ASCR's search site allows you to search specialties that include cataract, cornea, general or pediatric ophthalmology, glaucoma, LASEK, LASIK, oculoplastic, refractive, or retina.

Some highly skilled specialists in private practices are not associated with universities or medical schools. If, however, you haven't been able to get a recommendation and you are searching for a good doctor for follow-up or first-time care, it can be a good idea to begin your search by first looking at teaching hospitals or other academic medical centers. These institutions often are on the cutting edge of eye care, and doctors associated with them have a good chance of being familiar with the latest developments in their field.

Advertisements versus Personal and Professional Referrals

Some people rely solely on advertisements from newspapers, magazines, Web sites, television or radio when choosing a surgeon to perform their eye surgery. Ads can be useful for alerting you to the presence of an eye surgery clinic in your area. They also may provide some information about pricing. But this, of course, isn't enough for you to make an informed, intelligent choice when selecting a doctor to operate on your eyes.

Ads are self-referrals and do not come with a recommendation from someone you trust who, in turn, trusts the doctor. Advertising should only add a name to your list of doctors to consider after you have evaluated them and the services they offer.

This applies to your choice of doctor for your second surgery or treatment as much as it applies to your choice of doctor to perform your first operation.

It may not be a good idea to travel far from home to have your first operation because it would be inconvenient returning to the physician if complications develop. If, however, you are not satisfied with the eye care specialists near you, you may want to consider this inconvenience if you can afford it. And if you have difficult-to-treat complications, you may have no choice but to travel to the doctor best qualified to treat them. If the follow-up treatment specialist you travel to see has the experience and credentials that make her the best choice for dealing with your complaint, the potential benefits would probably outweigh the inconvenience of travel.

Online Sources for Treating Postsurgical Complications

If you are using online sources and search engines to compile a list of doctors for your consideration, make a list of your symptoms and complaints. Some search terms that describe eye care professionals who specialize in treating postsurgical complications include ophthalmology second opinion, dry eye or eyes, dry eye treatment, postrefractive surgery complications, refractive cornea surgery complications, postsurgical corneas, specialty contact lenses, postsurgical contact lenses, postsurgical corneal rehabilitation, specialty contact lens fitting, RGP, Z-Wave lenses, MacroLens and scleral lens.

Ophthalmologist-Recommended Hospitals

US News and World Report polled ophthalmologists to recommend hospitals providing treatment in their field. The following hospitals had "the highest recommendations from specialists in ophthalmology for challenging cases and procedures":

- Bascom Palmer Eye Institute at the University of Miami
  Locations in Miami, Naples, Plantation, and Palm Beach
  888-845-0002
  www.bpei.med.miami.edu
- Wilmer Eye Institute, Johns Hopkins Hospital
  600 North Wolfe Street
  Baltimore, MD 21287
  800-215-6467
  www.hopkinsmedicine.org/wilmer
- Wills Eye Hospital
  840 Walnut Street
  Philadelphia, PA 19017
  215-928-3000
  www.willseye.org
- Massachusetts Eye and Ear Infirmary
  Massachusetts General Hospital
  243 Charles Street
  Boston, MA 02114
  617-523-7900
  www.masseyeandear.org

- Jules Stein Eye Institute
  UCLA Medical Center, Los Angeles
  100 Stein Plaza UCLA
  Los Angeles, CA 90095-7000
  310-825-5000
  www.jsei.org
- University of Iowa Hospitals and Clinics
  200 Hawkins Drive
  Iowa City, IA 52242
  319-356-1616
  www.webeye.opth.viowa.edu
- Duke University Medical Center
  Duke Eye Center
  DUMC 3802
  Durham, NC 27710
  800-422-1575
  www.dukehealth.org/eye_center
- Doheny Eye Institute
  USC University Hospital
  323-442-7100
  www.doheny.org
- Emory University Hospital
  1364 Clifton Road
  Atlanta, GA 30322
  800-75-EMORY
  www.emoryhealthcare.org
- University of California
  San Francisco Medical Center
  500 Parnassus Avenue
  San Francisco, CA 94143
  888-689-UCSF
  referral.center@ucsfmedctr.org
  www.ucsfhealth.org
- Cleveland Clinic Cole Eye Institute
  9500 Euclid Avenue
  Cleveland, OH 44195
  800-223-2273
  www.clevelandclinic.org

- Mayo Clinic
  200 First Street Southwest
  Rochester, MN 55905
  507-284-2511
  www.mayoclinic.org/rochester/
- Cullen Eye Institute
  Methodist Hospital
  7200B Cambridge
  Houston, TX 77030
  713-798-6100
  www.bcm.edu/eye/
- Barnes-Jewish Hospital/Washington University
  1 Barnes-Jewish Hospital Plaza
  St. Louis, MO 63110
  314-747-3000
  www.barnesjewish.org
- New York Eye and Ear Infirmary
  310 East 14th Street
  New York, NY 10003
  212-979-4000
  www.nyee.edu
- W.K. Kellogg Eye Center
  University of Michigan
  1000 Wall Street
  Ann Arbor, MI 48105
  734-763-8122
  www.kellogg.umich.edu
- University of Illinois Medical Center
  1740 West Taylor Street
  Chicago, IL 60612
  866-600-CARE
  www.med.umich.edu

The Vision Surgery Rehab Network (www.visionsurgeryrehab.org/vsrnnetwork.html) also maintains a list of healthcare providers offering services for postsurgical complications. This site may be able to refer you to someone closer to you. You can try them by e-mailing info@vision surgeryrehab.org or by leaving a message on their toll-free voice-messaging system at 877-666-8776.

If you don't have any referrals for an appropriate doctor, you might consider using a service, such as MDNationwide.org (www.mdnation wide.org/; telephone toll-free 877-242-8556), a company that provides background information on physicians. For $9.99 it provides a statewide list of medical specialists it considers worthy of recommendation based on their credentials. The price of recommendations for doctors across the country is $24.95.

How to Learn About a Doctor's Background

With a good recommendation from another eye care provider, friend, or acquaintance, there may be no reason to research a physician's background. But if you don't have such a referral and you are comparing prospective healthcare providers, resources are available to provide information that may help you choose.

The Better Business Bureau (www.bbb.org/us/Find-Business-Reviews) may be able to tell you if there have been any complaints registered against a particular business. It is important to remember that anyone can register a complaint and that it is usually necessary to hear both sides of a story before drawing any conclusions. The same advice applies to lawsuits. Physicians can be sued without good cause. If, however, you discover a pattern of complaints or multiple lawsuits, it is a sign that you should investigate carefully before you choose that physician.

Sources of Information about Doctors

The American Board of Medical Specialties (ABMS), 222 North LaSalle Street, Suite 1500, Chicago, IL 60601, confirms ophthalmologist board certifications (or other medical specialists) for free online (www.abms.org) or by toll-free phone at 866-ASK-ABMS (275-2267). The ABMS does not charge to tell you whether a physician is board-certified, but it does not recommend doctors or provide other information.

To find information about a doctor from your state medical board, locate the board's contact information on the Web site of the FSMB (Federation of State Medical Boards): (www.fsmb.org/directory_smb.html). The directory of state medical boards is listed on the FSMB's public services tab.

The FSMB itself is a good source of background information about a physician you are considering. For a fee of $9.95, its DocInfo page (www.docinfo.org) provides a profile of medical doctors, osteopathic physicians, and most physician assistants who are licensed to practice in the United States. The profile promises to include records of disciplinary action by state medical boards, educational history, board certification, licenses in any states, and whether or not the person has used another name in the past. It does not include information about insurance-related legal issues such as lawsuits or medical malpractice claims or settlements. This information is available from court records and some-times from the profiles you can purchase from for-profit businesses (such as those listed at the end of this chapter) that provide background information about physicians and other professionals.

The "DoctorFinder" service of American Medical Association (AMA) (webapps.ama-assn.org/doctorfinder/html/patient.html) pro-vides very basic information about more than 814,000 MDs and ODs in the United States. The site provides more information concerning education, office hours, and insurance coverage, for example, if the physician is an AMA member. The same AMA Web site also provides a list of all state medical societies, which are other potential sources of information for you to consider.

Researching a prospective healthcare provider's background never guarantees first-rate, successful care, but it helps to avoid inexperienced and/or incompetent care.

Physician Background Checks for a Fee

Several companies keep up-to-date records about physicians cur-rently practicing medicine in all disciplines. For a fee starting at $20, these for-profit investigators provide information about a doctor's edu-cation, medical specialties, certifications, and professional membership affiliation. Some include other relevant information, such as a doctor's history of honors, awards, academic affiliations, and publications as well as contact information. MDNationwide.org (www.mdnation-wide.org; telephone toll-free 877-242-8556) charges $19.95 for this serv-ice, which includes past or pending disciplinary investigations.

USARecordsSearch (www.investigateyourdoctor.com/; telephone 818-745-1212) also provides background information on professionals for a fee ($35).

Chapter Fourteen

Dealing with Depression Caused by Vision Loss

It's normal to experience a low mood occasionally and not know precisely why. It also is completely natural to feel sad if you experience an obvious setback or an unpleasant or disturbing event. The feelings that accompany the loss of someone close, or something dear, to you are not symptoms of clinical depression; they are appropriate expressions of sadness, grief, mourning, or bereavement. These feelings only become symptoms of depression if they linger for weeks or months, and if they are more severe than they are for most people undergoing the same experience.

Big setbacks can, however, contribute to depression in susceptible individuals. For example, more than half of the people who lost their homes due to foreclosure experienced depression, and 37 percent experienced major depression, according to an August 2009 report in the *American Journal of Public Health*. It's not difficult to predict that other types of significant setbacks, including impaired vision, could be a risk factor for developing serious depression.

Major depression, or major depressive disorder, is the most serious form of this type of mood disorder. It is characterized by multiple symptoms, described later in this chapter, that result in an inability to function in all aspects of life. Some people have one episode of major depression, while others have more than one. Some people may require long-term treatment to prevent recurring episodes.

A less disabling form of depression is sometimes called mild, minor, or moderate depression, but it is mild, minor, or moderate only in the sense that it is not completely debilitating. Clinically it is called dysthymia. While its symptoms last a long time, they do not prevent complete functioning in day-to-day activities. They do, however, prevent people from functioning at a high level and from experiencing a fulfilling life.

Depression is more than a mental or psychological condition. It is a medical condition that interferes with your ability to feel satisfaction or pleasure. It prevents you from experiencing a sense of accomplishment.

It can also threaten your physical health, because its symptoms often include a significant increase or decrease in eating and sleeping.

Clinical depression affects your self-image and self-confidence, your thoughts, and your behavior. Untreated, it can lead to physical decline and suicide. It needs to be treated.

The condition is hardly rare: Nearly 21 million adults in the United States have some form of depression in any given year. In 2005, one in ten people in the United States took an antidepressant medication, according to a study published in the *Archives of General Psychiatry*.

Major depressive disorders may be increasing. Recent surveys indicate that cases of major depression in adults increased from a little more than 3 percent in 1991 to 1992 to a little more than 7 percent a decade later. In fact, the World Health Organization claims that depression disables more people around the world than any other medical condition. If you suffer from depression because your vision has become impaired, and there appears to be no way to restore your sight, it is not your fault. And according to the reports of many patients and doctors, it is not unusual for you to develop depression in response to permanent changes in your ability to see clearly.

There is, however, good news associated with this common threat to health: depression is often highly treatable. Most cases are mild or moderate and may respond to psychotherapy alone. In cases of severe depression, antidepressant medications, prescribed and monitored by a physician, provide a highly effective treatment often in combination with psychotherapy.

The Link Between Impaired Vision and Depression

One out of every three people with visual impairments showed signs of depression serious enough to interfere with normal, daily activities for two weeks or more, according to a study conducted by the Arlene R. Gordon Research Institute of Lighthouse International.

The magnitude of the impact of impaired vision on people's lives is reflected in a 2005 *American Journal of Geriatric Psychiatry* article: More than a quarter of older adults who recognized the need for vision rehabilitation suffered from mild depression, while 7 percent suffered from major depression. If these figures are generally applicable to adults whose vision has become impaired, then the rate of depression in this population is greater than it is in the general population.

Christie Sindt, OD, optometrist, and associate professor of clinical ophthalmology at the University of Iowa in Iowa City, Iowa, says that depression is definitely a problem among people who live with serious complications following refractive eye surgery.[1] In fact, she maintains that any person with a chronic vision problem is vulnerable to depression. And LASIK patients whose vision is worse after surgery bear an additional burden, according to Sindt: they feel remorse on top of depression, because they voluntarily submitted to the procedure that resulted in their discomfort and loss of vision.

"Anybody who suffers from chronic eye pain or chronic vision loss can suffer from depression," says Sindt, who is also the director of the Contact Lens Clinic in the Department of Ophthalmology and Visual Sciences at University of Iowa Hospitals and Clinics, in the March 2008 issue of *University of Iowa Healthcare Today*. "So this isn't exclusive to people with postrefractive surgery problems. It can happen when somebody has paid for a procedure as opposed to having a disease or an accident. When somebody has paid for a procedure, not only do they have to learn to adjust and live with their new vision or the pain in their eyes, they also have to learn to forgive themselves for having undergone a procedure that was elective. And for some people—it's very difficult for them to forgive themselves."

Chronic unrelenting pain, especially chronic eye pain, can lead to depression. Eye pain can be so debilitating that some patients seek removal of the entire eye. A painful blind eye is a standard indication for a procedure called enucleation, in which the whole eye, except for the eye muscles, is removed.

To many people, it is not surprising that a failed surgery leading to decreased vision accompanied with pain leads to depression. This can happen not only with refractive surgery but any of the eye surgeries.

Other professionals who treat patients with vision loss agree. Lylas G. Mogk, MD, told listeners at the March 25, 2004, Pfizer Ophthalmology Therapeutic Area Conference that vision loss is associated with more depression than just about any other condition, including heart disease, lung disease, and even cancer. "As research is now proving to us," he said, "depression with adult-onset vision loss is not correlated to age, sex, marital status, living situation, or degree of vision loss itself. It is correlated almost exclusively with functional capacity. If you can still do the things you want to do, you are far less likely to become depressed. This makes intuitive sense if you keep in mind that blind people across the country lead full lives without depression. But what these results also tell us is that a little...vision loss can impact function tremendously, so visual rehabilitation early on is crucial."

Do Irreparable Complications of LASIK Surgery Increase the Risk of Depression?

While there is little doubt that vision impairment is associated with an increased risk of depression,[2] it is harder to find convincing data showing that unsuccessful LASIK surgery in particular results in a higher risk of depression. There are several personal accounts of this happening, and critics of the procedure have attributed several suicides to unsuccessful refractive eye surgery. But these anecdotal accounts don't convince most eye care professionals.

Some skeptics of the association between unsuccessful LASIK surgery and depression contend that patients who develop depression were probably predisposed to the condition before their surgery. Dr. Steven C. Schallhorn, for example, former head of the Navy Refractive Surgery Center in San Diego, told a reporter[1] that no cause-and-effect relationship exists between LASIK complications and depression.

Although the FDA plans to gather definitive data to determine the frequency and effect of LASIK surgery complications on patients' quality of life, including incidents of depression, at this time there is little scientifically reliable proof of a connection. Lack of proof does not mean there is no association between LASIK complications and depression, of course; it just means the testimony of individuals who report problems remain only anecdotal accounts. Scientific progress and the accompanying changes it can bring require evidence gathered under controlled conditions; personal accounts, while telling, are not scientific proof of the existence of a link. Since millions of people undergo LASIK and other eye surgery with good results, the negative experiences of a few are dismissed by skeptics, who maintain that when depression does develop in a patient, it is because the patient was predisposed to developing the disorder even before undergoing surgery. Obviously, people with a history of depression should be screened very carefully before undergoing a medically unnecessary procedure that has even a small chance of complications.

On the other hand, the close link between vision loss in general and depression strongly suggests that a link between unsuccessful LASIK surgery and depression is highly likely.

Your Response to Vision Loss

If you have experienced depression in the past, you have a greater chance of developing depression in response to loss of vision. Other factors reflecting your quality of life can also affect your risk of developing depression. These include social isolation, including lack of friends and family, other health problems, and a lack of confidence in your ability to handle life-changing challenges.

The best predictor of whether vision loss will result in depression is not how much vision has been lost, but how the change in vision affects your ability to do what you did before your eyesight became impaired. In other words, if you can manage to do most of what you could do before your loss of vision, you are less likely to become depressed. Obviously many people with severe vision loss, even complete blindness, overcome the handicap and learn to function well without suffering from permanent depression.

Successfully dealing with your depression increases the chances of participation in and benefit from rehabilitation therapy designed to help you function with vision loss. And learning to successfully tolerate and/or compensate for vision loss may lessen the seriousness of your depression.

We live in a society geared toward youthful individuals. In fact, we live in a society that is even more geared toward sighted individuals. Impaired vision affects not only your ability to function in your professional and private lives; it also affects your self-image and relationship to others, because we live in communities in which it is assumed that everyone can see well. When you lose that ability, you are at risk of feeling cutoff from others.

Anger

The realization that vision impairment may be permanent can produce feelings of frustration with the inability to see as well as you could before surgery, anger over what has happened, and resentment at the medical profession and even with people who have had successful eye surgery. As mentioned, these feelings are natural responses to learning that your visual impairment—induced by elective surgery—cannot be corrected. At some point, however, you must accept your loss and resolve to compensate for it and function as well as you can in order to successfully adjust to your new circumstances.

If you fail to accept the setback and the limitations it imposes on you, it can result in a lower quality of life than if you made a sincere effort to adjust to the discomfort and concentrate on what you can do. Even in cases of severe pain, such as from extremely dry eyes, there are treatments including contact lenses, goggles, and preservative-free lubricating eyedrops that have been shown to relieve the discomfort enough to allow individuals to concentrate on activities that distract them from their visual loss and lessen chances of being incapacitated by depression.

Remorse

If elective surgery has made your vision worse, regret and remorse at having made the decision to undergo the procedure is obviously a normal response. Mourning over your loss of vision is expected. If, however, after a several weeks, you have not resolved to either continue seeking treatment or sought help in learning to live with your visual impairment through rehabilitative therapy, you might benefit from talking to a professional who can help you adjust to the quality of vision you still have. If you continue to show signs of lack of motivation, exhaustion, and feelings of hopelessness and worthlessness, you should seek treatment from a qualified doctor, such as a psychologist or psychiatrist.

Dealing with Depression

No set number or array of symptoms characterizes depression. They can vary from person to person. Some symptoms may appear as others fade, and they may last for different periods of time. It is the pattern of changes and how they affect your mood and life that should alert you to the possibility that you could be clinically depressed and could benefit from treatment.

Dealing with Hopelessness and Helplessness

Two facts may help you overcome feelings of helplessness. First, medical research does not stop. It may progress quickly in some areas and slowly in others, but there is always the chance that new lenses and new medical treatments may be developed to help you. Second, rehabilitative therapy for impaired vision has helped thousands of people and may help you concentrate on what you can do rather than only mourn the vision you have lost.

Dealing with Feelings of Worthlessness and Inferiority

Common to depression, these feelings are more symptoms of the disease than they are an accurate reflection of your situation. These feelings may be effectively eliminated by medical treatment.

Dealing with Exhaustion and Lack of Motivation

These symptoms of depression respond remarkably well to medical treatment and therapy. It is not likely for serious depression to subside by itself. With treatment, however, it can begin to improve in a matter of weeks. Improvement may begin slowly, but recovery is common with treatment.

Recognizing the Signs of Depression

If you or someone you care about has experienced at least two weeks of constant, daylong periods of depressed mood or loss of interest (the top two symptoms listed in the sidebar on this page) as well as at least four of the other signs, it is important to see a psychologist or psychiatrist who is qualified to diagnose mood disorders. A physical exam can identify or rule out metabolic or other physical conditions that might cause or contribute to the symptoms. If the cause does turn out to be a major depressive disorder, the physician may treat it with a combination of medication and psychotherapy. It is very important that depressive disorders are treated. It is unsafe to assume a spontaneous recovery. Depression can be a life-threatening condition, but it is one that often responds well to treatment.

Do You Have Symptoms of Depression?

The National Institute of Mental Health advises that you may be suffering from depression if you experience the following symptoms:
- persistent sad, anxious, depressed, or "empty" mood
- loss of interest or pleasure in previously enjoyed hobbies and activities
- feelings of hopelessness or pessimism
- feelings of guilt, worthlessness, or helplessness
- decreased energy, fatigue, or feeling "slowed down"
- difficulty concentrating, remembering, and making decisions

- trouble sleeping, early-morning awakening, or oversleeping
- appetite and/or weight changes
- thoughts of death or suicide or suicide attempts
- restlessness or irritability
- persistent physical symptoms, such as headaches, digestive disorders, and chronic pain that do not respond to routine treatment

Source: National Institute of Mental Health, Depression: A Treatable Illness Fact Sheet

If you have one of the first two symptoms on the above list but fewer than five total symptoms over the course of at least two weeks, you could have a mild or minor depressive disorder. In fact, minor depression is more common than major depressive disorders; more people with vision impairment suffer from minor depression than major depression. Nevertheless, the symptoms can significantly lower your quality of life and even make it more difficult to learn how to cope with vision loss. Minor depression can also respond well to treatment.

Sources of Help

The eye care professionals you see as you seek medical treatment for your eyes (eye surgeons and other ophthalmologists and optometrists) are not trained as psychologists or psychiatrists; it is not their job to counsel you or provide therapy. Professional eye care providers, especially those with medical degrees, however, should be able to recognize obvious signs of depression. They should be able to refer you to someone trained in psychology or psychiatry. Nevertheless, you may have to recognize depression in yourself and seek help from a mental health professional if dealing with your visual problem is seriously undermining the quality of your life.

Often the best way to find someone to help you treat depression is to get a referral from a friend, family member, acquaintance, or family doctor. If no one you know can recommend a good therapist or doctor, you might contact a local community mental health center (CMHCs) that provides outpatient services. To locate one near you, contact the Substance Abuse and Mental Health Service Administration's Mental Health Information Center. The 24-hour referral telephone number is 800-662-HELP (800-662-4357). You can also e-mail nmhic-info@samhsa.hhs.gov, visit the Mental Health Services Locator Web site at mentalhealth.samhsa.gov/databases, or write to PO Box 42557, Washington, DC 20015.

Another source of information and referrals to local mental health services is The National Suicide Prevention Lifeline (800-273-TALK [8255]). It offers 24-hour advice on many topics concerning mental health as well as suicide.

The National Institute of Mental Health suggests the following resources for people who want help dealing with depression:
- mental health specialists, such as psychiatrists, psychologists, social workers, or mental health counselors
- health maintenance organizations
- community mental health centers
- hospital psychiatry departments and outpatient clinics
- mental health programs at universities or medical schools
- state hospital outpatient clinics
- family services, social agencies, or clergy
- peer support groups
- private clinics and facilities
- employee assistance programs
- local medical and/or psychiatric societies

You can also check the phone book under headings such as mental health, health, social services, hotlines, or physicians for phone numbers and addresses. An emergency room doctor also can provide temporary help and can tell you where and how to get further help.

Resources for Depression Treatment

These organizations provide useful information and advice concerning treatment for depression:
- The National Library of Medicine's Medline Plus
  www.nlm.nih.gov/medlineplus/depression.html
- National Institute of Mental Health
  Science Writing, Press & Dissemination Branch
  6001 Executive Boulevard, Room 8184 MSC 9663
  Bethesda, MD 20892-9663

866-615-6464
E-mail: nimhinfo@nih.gov
www.nimh.nih.gov
Web site devoted to depression:
www.nimh.nih.gov/health/topics/depression/index.
shtml

- National Alliance for the Mentally Ill
3803 North Fairfax Drive, Suite 100
Arlington, VA 22203
703-524-7600
Information Helpline: 800-950-6264
www.nami.org
Web site devoted to depression:
www.nami.org/Template.cfm?Section=depression
- National Depressive and Manic Depressive
Association
730 North Franklin, Suite 501
Chicago, IL 60601
800-826-3632
www.ndmda.org
- Mental Health America
2000 North Beauregard Street, 6th Floor
Alexandria, VA 22311
800-969-6642
www.nmha.org

Treating Depression

It might seem obvious to you that any feelings of depression you have are completely related to problems with your vision. Although you may be right, it is still necessary to get a thorough, complete physical examination to rule out other medical conditions (such as a problem with your thyroid or even an infection, for example) that might account for or contribute to symptoms of depression.

Treatment for depression can begin after a proper diagnosis by a mental health professional. It can follow different courses, which is determined by the severity of your symptoms, your state of health, and your personal preferences.

Depression is like many other illnesses; it is often easier to treat in its early stages. Early treatment can head off more severe symptoms and decrease the chances of experiencing recurring bouts of depression.

You and your doctor or therapist can choose from a variety of medications and psychotherapies. For some individuals, symptoms may improve with the help of a psychotherapist alone. Others may get relief with minimal therapy and short-term medication. Therapy for depression may be relatively short-term, lasting only months, or, depending on the person and the degree of depression, it may continue for life. A combination of antidepressant medications and some type of talk therapy has been shown to be particularly effective in treating severe cases of illness. These combinations of treatment options allow most people to overcome depression when the right treatment plan is found and followed.

Medications

Depression is linked to changes in the function of chemical messengers called neurotransmitters in the brain. These brain chemicals—serotonin, norepinephrine, and dopamine—influence mood and feelings. Antidepressant medications compensate for errors in the functioning of one or more of these neurotransmitter systems.

Some antidepressants increase levels of serotonin by preventing the neurotransmitter from being removed from its site of action in the brain. These selective serotonin reuptake inhibitors (SSRIs), including Prozac, Celexa, and Zoloft, are particularly popular antidepressants today, but other classes of antidepressants are available if you don't respond well to SSRIs. Effexor, for instance, is a serotonin and norepinephrine reuptake inhibitor (SNRI). Older types of antidepressants inhibit an enzyme called monoamine oxidase (MAO) and are called MAO inhibitors (MAOIs). Other medications still used to treat depression are tricyclic antidepressants, which are named for their chemical structure. Your doctor can recommend a wide variety of medications based on your needs, responses, and preferences.

Many doctors today are prescribing a second medication along with one of the above antidepressants. The combination of this add-on medication, such as Abilify and a main antidepressant, such as Effexor XR, Lexapro, Paxil CR, Zoloft, or Prozac, has been shown to improve depressive symptoms even more than prescriptions of single antidepressants.

Keep in Mind When Starting an Antidepressant...

It is important that your doctor is familiar with the properties of any medication she prescribes for you. She should explain the expected benefits, limitations and side effects. It may be necessary to try more than one antidepressant before you and your doctor find one that works best. A qualified professional is aware of, and will warn you about, side effects and dietary restrictions, if any, that are important to follow while you are taking certain medications. And be wary of a physician who fails to take a thorough medical history and/or writes you a prescription and sends you on your way without discussing the advisability and options of combining drug treatment with psychotherapy.

While the different classes of antidepressants vary widely in structure and the way they work in the brain, they all have something in common: it takes a while before they have a noticeable effect on your mood. Their full effects may not be felt for several weeks or longer. It is during this time that you must rely on yourself and your psychotherapist, if you have one, to deal with your depression.

Tips for Managing Depression While Beginning Treatment

During the lag between beginning treatment for depression and relief of symptoms, it important to fight the despair that accompanies the mood disorder. The National Institute of Mental Health (NIMH) offers the following advice:

"If you have depression, you may feel exhausted, helpless, and hopeless. It may be extremely difficult to take any action to help yourself. But it is important to realize that these feelings are part of the depression and do not accurately reflect actual circumstances. As you begin to recognize your depression and begin treatment, negative thinking will fade."

To help yourself, the NIMH has some suggestions:

- Engage in mild activity or exercise. Listen to music, or engage in other activities that you once enjoyed. Participate in religious, social, or other activities.
- Set realistic goals for yourself.
- Break up large tasks into small ones, set some priorities, and do what you can as you can.
- Try to spend time with other people and confide in a trusted friend or relative. Try not to isolate yourself, and let others help you.
- Expect your mood to improve gradually, not immediately. Do not expect to suddenly "snap out of" your depression. Often during treatment for depression, sleep and appetite improves before your depressed mood lifts.
- Postpone important decisions, such as getting married or divorced or changing jobs, until you feel better. Discuss decisions with others who know you well and have a more objective view of your situation.
- Remember that positive thinking replaces negative thoughts as your depression responds to treatment.

Enlist help to establish a plan to locate and consult with specialists who treat the specific problem or problems that have impaired your vision. If you have tried or benefited from such treatment and are still left with uncorrectable visual impairment, enlist help to formulate a plan to get all the benefits you can from rehabilitative therapy, which may increase your ability to compensate for your loss and relieve your distress as much as possible.

Low Vision Centers may be very helpful to you if your vision is severely impaired.[3] They have a variety of tools and aids that can magnify, or illuminate, your visual environment to make your tasks easier. Initially you receive a comprehensive eye evaluation, and then you will be introduced to the various tools that may make your visual tasks easier. You can look up these centers in the yellow pages under "low vision," or ask an eye care professional for a reference.

After medications begin to relieve depression, it is also important that you do not stop taking them on your own, without the supervision of your doctor. The best way to discontinue many medications is to gradually reduce the dose under a physician's direction.

Psychotherapy

Often called talk therapy, psychotherapy may benefit some individuals in as few as two and a half to five months, while others need more time. The length is determined by the severity of the depression and the patient's response. In cases of mild depression, psychotherapy alone may be enough to overcome the problem.

Some types of psychotherapy are more effective for treating depression than others. Cognitive–behavioral therapy (CBT) in particular has been shown in well-controlled studies to help overcome mood disorders.

Minor or moderate depression often responds particularly well to CBT; in some cases it works even in the absence of antidepressant medications. It has also been shown to be effective when given in combination with antidepressants. Its effectiveness seems to lie in its ability to change thought patterns, making them less negative. This, in turn, changes how an individual regards his circumstances and prospects for a meaningful life. While impaired vision may be a key factor in the cause of the depression, it is possible to change how a person reacts to this disturbing challenge. Restructuring this response can help prevent worsening of the depression. A good CBT therapist can help you develop new, more positive ways of thinking, behaving, and feeling as you cope with visual impairment.

Another type of therapy to be useful in treating depression is interpersonal therapy (IPT). This type of talk therapy is most often used with individuals who have dysthymia, a mild but long-lasting type of depression. It is particularly suited for helping people deal with interpersonal relationships. This could be a factor if vision impairment is causing stress in a relationship.

Chapter Fifteen

Benefits of Low-Vision Rehabilitation

If your vision can't be improved with glasses, contacts, surgery, or medication—and it prevents you from carrying out and enjoying the usual activities of your daily life—you might benefit from low-vision rehabilitation. Statistics on the number of people dealing with low vision vary, depending on the definition of low vision. In 2006, the estimated number of adults with vision problems that could not be corrected with contact lenses or glasses ranged from 3 million to 19 million.

Age-related macular degeneration may be responsible for half of all cases of low vision in this country. The majority of the remaining cases are due to diabetic retinopathy, glaucoma, retinitis pigmentosa (night blindness), or cataracts. Other diseases and injuries account for the rest. If you are one of the rare persons whose low vision can be traced to complications from eye surgery, you may still benefit from the low-vision rehabilitation services that have evolved in response to needs created by the most common eye diseases.

Seeing double or distorted images, having visual acuity worse than 20/70, having a limited visual field, and not being able to detect contrasts or tolerate light can all qualify as low vision—as long as the problem significantly hinders your ability to perform the normal activities of daily living. Some people have combinations of such problems.

No matter what the cause or nature of your visual impairment, don't assume you can't improve your situation even if the problem cannot be reversed by current medical treatments. You may not be able to regain your lost vision, but you may be able to compensate for some of the problems the loss causes you. You may be able to function on a much higher level than you thought. The American Academy of Ophthalmology (AAO) suggests the sooner you start vision rehabilitation after developing untreatable vision problems, the better.

Successful vision rehabilitation may allow you to regain self-confidence and make the most of your remaining sight by stressing practical solutions to problems that hinder your ability to perform activities that are part of daily living, such as reading, driving, maintaining a home, running errands outside the home, caring for yourself, and taking part in social and recreational pastimes.

The Best Treatment Now and in the Future

A good doctor makes certain that your vision impairment is indeed untreatable and permanent. Make sure the doctors you consult are familiar with cutting-edge treatments, including the latest in therapeutic contact lenses, surgical options, and medications. New treatments and new lenses that become available in the future may help relieve your symptoms.

Steps to Take If Your Low-Vision Condition Seems to Be Permanent

If your problems are the result of LASIK or other eye surgeries, here are three potentially valuable things to do if you have not been able to find relief:

- Confirm that you have received the best treatment and advice from the doctors you have consulted. This can be done by getting second and third opinions, if necessary, and educating yourself about the nature of your condition.
- Get help, if necessary, for any feelings of despair, hopelessness, or depression. Progress toward this goal is necessary to get the most benefit from the vision rehabilitation.
- Develop coping strategies and take advantage of any suggestions, ideas, training, and compensatory skills you can develop independently or learn by attending low- or impaired-vision rehabilitation programs.

Preparing to Cope

To build a life around your visual limitations, you first have to accept what has changed in your life. Once you have accepted the limitations of your vision, you can concentrate on the activities you can do and begin to develop approaches for compensating for activities you cannot do. It is important that you recognize that your impairment is something that must be overcome either by treatment or, if that is not possible, by changed behavior, adaptation, training, and the practice of new skills. Emphasize your remaining sight and remember that many people who lack sight altogether have successfully maximized their ability to live independently.

Depending on your symptoms, your vision may require major adjustments to your lifestyle. If, for example, your night vision has been affected severely, you may no longer be able to drive at night. Loss of freedom and being forced to give up previously routine activities can be depressing and demoralizing. This is why professional psychological help may be a crucial part of your rehabilitation. At the same time, rehabilitation therapists claim that progress made through low-vision rehabilitation itself contributes to improved morale and mood.

Taking Inventory of Your Needs

Even before you consult a low-vision rehabilitation specialist, note which of your activities are affected by your vision problem and which are not. What can you still do well? The answer may suggest strategies for coping with some of the tasks made more difficult or impossible by your visual loss.

What can you do less well? What specific tasks would you like to be able to do despite your impaired eyesight? An inventory aids in identifying goals and develop strategies to help you achieve them. Your optometrist or ophthalmologist can also help you engage in as many activities, and live your life as fully as your visual impairment allows.

After a thorough evaluation of your abilities, a low-vision specialist may be able to recommend and provide you with special equipment to help you adapt to living with impaired vision.

Your Low-Vision Rehab Examination and Therapeutic Plan

The condition of your eyes has a big influence on the type of rehabilitation that will help you most. Different diseases and injuries have different effects on the eye and its ability to function. Your low-vision assessment factors your medical history into a therapeutic plan to meet your visual needs and capabilities. Strategies and therapies for coping with your individual low-vision profile are developed and passed on to an eye care provider who will train you to make the most of your vision.

Common Areas of Concern Targeted in Low-Vision Therapeutic Plans

Vision rehabilitation specialists have considered and tested many ways to get around or compensate for different types of low-vision problems. And manufacturers of special low-vision products continue to develop and test new devices to aid those with low vision. These devices range from antiglare filters to state-of-the-art electronic cameras and sensors for improving people's ability to sense their surroundings despite serious visual disabilities.

Other vision rehabilitation services may help you learn to be more mobile, offer counseling, suggest ways to modify your home to make it easier to complete everyday tasks, and train you to use special adaptive aids and equipment.

The following are some examples of approaches used to restore independence and improve the lives of people with low vision. Since individual needs vary depending on the nature of each person's visual loss, these are only a sampling of potentially helpful aids and strategies. Vision rehabilitation specialists have many more techniques and approaches that they can recommend.

Reading

If magnification can help overcome your vision problem, you have a choice of assistive devices, ranging from magnifying eyeglasses to different types of stand-alone magnifiers.

Today, technology goes far beyond large-print books. Computers can be used to enlarge print, making it easier to read. Closed-circuit television or a video magnifier uses a video camera to send an image of a page to a big screen for easy reading. This approach also allows readers to adjust contrast in addition to magnifying letters and illustrations.

If magnification cannot help you, low-vision therapists may discuss using electronic reading machines and software that can scan printed material and read it aloud to you. Audio books, of course, are widely available on CD and in various electronic formats that can be played through MP3 players and iPods.

Patients with macular degeneration, for example, can often develop skills through rehabilitation training that allow them to continue reading as well as functioning at home and socializing.

Computers

Large-screen monitors are a start for many people with low vision, special software programs that can enlarge text on regular computer screens and even some that can read it to you are available. Voice-recognition software now enables users to speak commands and write "hands-free" with good accuracy. Standard keyboards can be replaced with versions equipped with large letters.

Other Close-Up Work or Near Vision

Large-print versions of many types of printed material besides books, such as playing cards and labels, are available. Markers that produce wider lines may eliminate some problems created by writing with ordinary pens and pencils. And everyday household items are now available in versions that talk, including thermometers, time pieces, calculators, and bathroom scales.

How to Find Low-Vision and Rehabilitation Specialists and Programs

You can find low-vision and rehabilitation specialists by asking your ophthalmologist or optometrist to recommend some in your area. Also, be sure to visit Light House International's Web site (www.Light house.org). This private agency offers people with visual impairments information on professional services, research results, and up-to-date advice on methods for dealing with low vision. The Light House Web site includes a link labeled "Help Near You" that can direct you to support groups as well as professional vision rehabilitation services. You can also phone Light House International at 800-829-0500.

State Rehabilitation Agencies are listed on the Vision Aware Web site (www.vision aware.org).

Low Vision Centers are also listed by state on the American Macular Degeneration Foundation's Web site (www.macular.org/lowvis).

Distance Vision

The telescope has long been used to improve distance vision. Telescopes designed to improve low vision can magnify distant objects up to 20 times their size. Now updated and improved, they can be mounted on eye glasses, called bioptics, for extended viewing, or they can be hand-held. Some eyeglass-mounted models are self-focusing, freeing users from having to manually adjust them as each new object is located.

Dealing with Glare and Light

Sometimes changes in the amount, type, and placement of lighting at home and in the workplace can make a big difference for people with low vision. Solutions as simple as wearing a visor or a hat may cut down on glare. Installing and relocating sources of illumination in the home and office can eliminate some problems and reduce irritation.

Filtering light through amber or yellow filters may reduce light scattering and other visual problems that cause lights to produce unwanted effects in certain situations. Filters made of other colors have other applications that are potentially useful for people bothered by glare or poor contrast imaging.

Traveling

There is no reason to be housebound because you have developed low vision. This attitude may be related to depression, embarrassment, or fear of getting lost. A mobility or orientation specialist can give you the skills to move freely on your own in familiar territory.

Social Support

Another benefit of vision rehabilitation is the opportunity it offers you to spend time with people who understand what you struggle with every day. They understand the stress and frustrations associated with having impaired vision. The same benefit may be found in support groups such as those compiled by Light House International (www.Lighthouse.org).

Informed Consent for LASIK

This modified example of an informed consent form is reprinted with permission of the Opthalmic Mutual Insurance Company.

This information is being provided to you so that you can make an informed decision about the use of a device known as a microkeratome, combined with the use of a device known as an excimer laser, to perform LASIK. LASIK is one of a number of alternatives for correcting nearsightedness, farsightedness, and astigmatism. In LASIK, the microkeratome is used to shave the cornea to create a flap. Then the flap is opened like the page of a book to expose tissue just below the cornea's surface. Next, the excimer laser is used to remove ultrathin layers from the cornea to reshape it to reduce nearsightedness. Finally, the flap is returned to its original position, without sutures.

LASIK is an elective procedure: there is no emergency condition or other reason that requires or demands that you have it performed. You could continue wearing contact lenses or glasses and have adequate visual acuity. This procedure, like all surgery, presents some risks, many of which are listed below. You should also understand that there may be other risks not known to your doctor, which may become known later. Despite the best of care, complications and side effects may occur; should this happen in your case, the result might be affected even to the extent of making your vision worse.

Alternatives to LASIK

If you decide not to have LASIK, your nearsightedness, farsightedness, or astigmatism can be corrected via other methods. These alternatives include, among others, eyeglasses, contact lenses, and other refractive surgical procedures.

Patient Consent

In giving my permission for LASIK, I understand the following: The long-term risks and effects of LASIK are unknown. I have received no guarantee as to the success of my particular case. I understand that the following risks are associated with the procedure:

Vision-Threatening Complications

1. I understand that the microkeratome or the excimer laser could malfunction, requiring the procedure to be stopped before completion. Depending on the type of malfunction, this may or may not be accompanied by visual loss.
2. I understand that, in using the microkeratome, instead of making a flap, an entire portion of the central cornea could be cut off and very rarely could be lost. If preserved, I understand that my doctor would put this tissue back on the eye after the laser treatment, using sutures, according to the automated lamellar keratoplasty (ALK) procedure method. It is also possible that the flap incision could result in an incomplete flap or a flap that is too thin. If this happens, it is likely that the laser part of the procedure will have to be postponed until the cornea has a chance to heal sufficiently to try to create the flap again.
3. I understand that irregular healing of the flap could result in a distorted cornea. This would mean that glasses or contact lenses may not correct my vision to the level possible before undergoing LASIK. If this distortion in vision is severe, a partial or complete corneal transplant might be necessary to repair the cornea.
4. I understand that it is possible a perforation of the cornea could occur, causing devastating complications, including loss of some or all of my vision. This could also be caused by an internal or external eye infection that could not be controlled with antibiotics or other means.
5. I understand that mild or severe infection is possible. Mild infection can usually be treated with antibiotics and usually does not lead to permanent visual loss. Severe infection, even if successfully treated with antibiotics, could lead to permanent scarring and loss of vision that may require corrective laser surgery or, if very severe, corneal transplantation or even loss of the eye.

6. I understand that I could develop keratoconus. Keratoconus is a degenerative corneal disease affecting vision that occurs in approximately 1/2000 in the general population. While there are several tests that suggest which patients might be at risk, this condition can develop in patients who have normal preoperative topography (a map of the cornea obtained before surgery) and pachymetry (corneal thickness measurement). Since keratoconus may occur on its own, there is no absolute test to ensure a patient will not develop keratoconus following laser vision correction. Severe keratoconus may need to be treated with a corneal transplant while mild keratoconus can be corrected by glasses or contact lenses.

7. I understand that other very rare complications threatening vision include, but are not limited to, corneal swelling, corneal thinning (ectasia), appearance of floaters and retinal detachment, hemorrhage, venous and arterial blockage, cataract formation, total blindness, and even loss of my eye.

Non-Vision-Threatening Side Effects

1. I understand that there may be increased sensitivity to light, glare, and fluctuations in the sharpness of vision. I understand these conditions usually occur during the normal stabilization period of from one to three months, but they may also be permanent.

2. I understand that there is an increased risk of eye irritation related to drying of the corneal surface following the LASIK procedure. These symptoms may be temporary or, on rare occasions, permanent, and may require frequent application of artificial tears and/or closure of the tear duct openings in the eyelid.

3. I understand that an overcorrection or under-correction could occur, causing me to become farsighted or nearsighted or increase my astigmatism and that this could be either permanent or treatable. I understand an overcorrection or under-correction is more likely in people over the age of 40 years and may require the use of glasses for reading or for distance vision some or all of the time.

4. After refractive surgery, a certain number of patients experience glare, a starburst or halo effect around lights, or other low-light vision problems that may interfere with the ability to drive at night or see well in dim light. The exact cause of these visual problems is not currently known; some ophthalmologists theorize that the risk

may be increased in patients with large pupils or high degrees of correction. For most patients, this is a temporary condition that diminishes with time or is correctable by wearing glasses at night or taking eyedrops. For some patients, however, these visual problems are permanent. I understand that my vision may not seem as sharp at night as during the day and that I may need to wear glasses at night or take eyedrops. I understand that it is not possible to predict whether I will experience these night vision or low-light problems, and that I may permanently lose the ability to drive at night or function in dim light because of them. I understand that I should not drive unless my vision is adequate.

5. I understand that I may not get a full correction from my LASIK procedure and this may require future enhancement procedures, such as more laser treatment or the use of glasses or contact lenses.

6. I understand that there may be a balance problem between my two eyes after LASIK has been performed on one eye and not the other. This phenomenon is called anisometropia. I understand this would cause eyestrain and make judging distance or depth perception more difficult. I understand that my first eye may take longer to heal than is usual, prolonging the time I could experience anisometropia.

7. I understand that, after LASIK, the eye may be more fragile to trauma from impact. Evidence has shown that, as with any scar, the corneal incision will not be as strong as the cornea originally was at that site. I understand that the treated eye, therefore, is somewhat more vulnerable to all varieties of injuries, at least for the first year following LASIK. I understand it would be advisable for me to wear protective eyewear when engaging in sports or other activities in which the possibility of a ball, projectile, elbow, fist, or other traumatizing object contacting the eye may be high.

8. I understand that there is a natural tendency of the eyelids to droop with age and that eye surgery may hasten this process.

9. I understand that there may be pain or a foreign-body sensation, particularly during the first 48 hours after surgery.

10. I understand that temporary glasses either for distance or reading may be necessary while healing occurs and that more than one pair of glasses may be needed.

11. I understand that the long-term effects of LASIK are unknown and that unforeseen complications or side effects could possibly occur.

12. I understand that visual acuity I initially gain from LASIK could

regress, and that my vision may go back to a level that may require glasses or contact lens use to see clearly.

13. I understand that the correction that I can expect to gain from LASIK may not be perfect. I understand that it is not realistic to expect that this procedure will result in perfect vision, at all times, under all circumstances, for the rest of my life. I understand that I may need glasses to refine my vision for some purposes requiring fine, detailed vision after some point in my life, and that this might occur soon after surgery or years later.

14. I understand that I may be given medication in conjunction with the procedure and that my eye may be patched afterward. I therefore understand that I must not drive the day of surgery and not until I am certain that my vision is adequate for driving.

15. I understand that if I currently need reading glasses, I will still likely need reading glasses after this treatment. It is possible that dependence on reading glasses may increase or that reading glasses may be required at an earlier age if I have this surgery.

16. Even 90 percent clarity of vision is still slightly blurry. Enhancement surgeries can be performed when vision is stable unless it is unwise or unsafe. If the enhancement is performed within the first six months following surgery, there generally is no need to make another cut with the microkeratome. The original flap can usually be lifted with specialized techniques. After six months of healing, a new LASIK incision may be required, incurring greater risk. In order to perform an enhancement surgery, there must be adequate tissue remaining. If there is inadequate tissue, it may not be possible to perform an enhancement. An assessment and consultation will be held with the surgeon, at which time the benefits and risks of an enhancement surgery will be discussed.

17. I understand that, as with all types of surgery, there is a possibility of complications due to anesthesia, drug reactions, or other factors that may involve other parts of my body. I understand that, since it is impossible to state every complication that may occur as a result of any surgery, the list of complications in this form may not be complete.

For Presbyopic Patients

Those requiring a separate prescription for reading:
The option of monovision has been discussed with my ophthalmologist.

Patient's Statement of Acceptance and Understanding

The details of the procedure known as LASIK have been presented to me in detail in this document and explained to me by my ophthalmologist. My ophthalmologist has answered all my questions to my satisfaction. I therefore consent to LASIK surgery on:

_____ Right eye _____ Left eye _____ Both eyes

I give permission for my ophthalmologist to record my procedure on video or photographic equipment for purposes of education, research, or training of other healthcare professionals. I also give my permission for my ophthalmologist to use data about my procedure and subsequent treatment to further understand LASIK. I understand that my name will remain confidential, unless I give subsequent written permission for it to be disclosed outside my ophthalmologist's office or the center where my LASIK procedure will be performed.

_____   _____
Patient Name   Date

_____   _____
Witness Name   Date

I have been offered a copy of this consent form (please initial) _____

Appendix C

Further Reading

Sophie J. Bakri, MD, (editor) *Mayo Clinic Guide to Better Vision* (Rochester, Minnesota: Mayo Clinic, 2007). Useful explanations and advice concerning many aspects of eye care, eye surgery, and eye diseases, including macular degeneration, glaucoma, cataracts, and diabetes.

Endnotes

Introduction
1. Peggy Peck, "FDA Advisers Find LASIK Safe but Oversold," MedPage Today, www.medpageto-day.com/Ophthalmology/LaserSurgery/9250 (April 25, 2008).
2. Sabine Vollmer, "Some Link Depression, Failed LASIK," The News & Observer, February 3, 2008.

Chapter Fourteen
1. ibid.
2. A. Horowitz, J.P. Reinhardt, and G. Kennedy, "Major and Subthreshold Depression among Older Adults Seeking Vision Rehabilitation Services," American Journal of Geriatric Psychiatry 13 (2005): 180-187.
3. A. Horowitz, M. Brennan, J.P. Reinhardt, and T. MacMillan, "The Impact of Assistive Device Use on Disability and Depression among Older Adults with Age-Related Vision Impairments," The Journals of Gerontology Series B: Psychological Sciences and Social Sciences 61 (2006): S274-S280.

Glossary

acuity (visual): The ability to perceive detail; the sharpness of one's vision.

amblyopia: Dim or reduced vision of unknown cause in an eye that appears normal. It is assumed to result from one eye getting less visual stimulation than the other during a critical period when the eye and brain establish connections. The connections from the amblyopic eye cause its images to be blurred. Often this eye turns outward as the brain ignores its input to avoid double vision.

anterior chamber: The front chamber of the eye bordered by the iris and pupil in back and the cornea in front. It is filled with aqueous humor.

aqueous humor: Nutritional fluid formed behind the iris in the ciliary body. It flows through the pupil to the front chamber of the eye and is filtered through the trabecular meshwork.

astigmatism: Uneven curvature of the cornea causing images to be unevenly focused on the retina. Occasionally a lack of symmetry on the surface of the lens is responsible for the same effect.

binocular vision: A visual benefit of anatomy in which the eyes are positioned in the front of the head and provide overlapping fields of vision. It results in good depth perception and better visual acuity.

blepharitis: A chronic, low-grade, noncontagious infection of the eyelid with accompanying inflammation.

branch retinal artery occlusion: A blockage in one of the arterial branches of the retina which results in decreased, or loss of, vision in the corresponding peripheral visual area. It is a warning sign of an increased risk of stroke. A thorough cardiac and cholesterol workup is advised.

branch retinal vein occlusion: A blood clot in a branch vein of the retina that can lead to blurred vision. Its effect can be permanent or sometimes temporary. High blood pressure is a risk factor.

cataract: Cloudiness or opacity of the eye's crystalline lens. Often the result of age, cataracts can also develop as a result of injury, disease or radiation. If it reduces vision to the point of interfering with a person's activities, it routinely is treated by removing the lens and replacing it with an artificial one.

central retinal artery occlusion: A blockage in the main artery of the eye with devastating irreversible loss of vision.

central retinal vein occlusion: A blood clot in a large main vein that drains blood from the eye resulting in sudden, painless blurred vision.

choroid: The middle layer of the eye. It has many blood vessels and contains pigments which help redirect light back onto the retina which lies above it.

closed angle glaucoma: A condition in which very high eye pressure builds up after the peripheral iris blocks drainage canals in the anterior chamber and prevents aqueous humor from draining.

ciliary body: A structure located behind the iris which produces aqueous humor.

conductive keratoplasty (CK): A treatment using heat to change the peripheral shape of the cornea. The resulting mild nearsightedness is intended to eliminate the need for reading glasses.

conjunctiva: The thin, clear mucus membrane covering the surface of the eye. It contains many blood vessels.

cornea: The clear, curved surface of the eye located in front of the retina, lens, and iris. It provides protection and much of the eye's focusing power.

diabetic retinopathy: Abnormal changes in the retina resulting from poorly controlled blood sugar. The swelling and bleeding that accompany it produce blurred vision.

dry eye (or dry eyes or dry eye syndrome): A collective term for the symptoms accompanying too little tears bathing the surface of the cornea. It produces sensations of scratchiness, redness, irritation, and light sensitivity.

epiretinal membrane: An abnormal membrane that grows on the surface of the retina which can cause blurred vision and image distortion.

esotropia: A condition in which the eyes turn inward. Commonly known as cross-eye, it is the result of a problem with eye muscles, or the nerves that control their actions.

exotropia: A condition in which the eyes turn outward. Commonly known as walleye, it is the result of a problem with eye muscles, or the nerves that control their actions.

Epi-LASEK: A type of refractive eye surgery that reshapes the cornea to correct near- or farsightedness. It differs from similar procedures by briefly presoaking the surface of the cornea with alcohol before a very sharp, precise instrument is used to slice a thin layer of the epithelium. This epithelial flap is moved aside and replaced after the cornea is reshaped using a laser.

Epi-LASIK: A type of refractive eye surgery that reshapes the cornea to correct near- or farsightedness. It uses a very sharp, precise instrument to slice a thin layer of the epithelium on the surface of the cornea to create a flap that is moved aside and replaced after the cornea is reshaped using a laser. Unlike epi-LASEK, no alcohol is used.

farsightedness: A condition in which an image is focused behind the retina, making near objects appear blurred and eventually far objects as well.

glaucoma: A family of eye diseases that cause optic nerve damage, resulting in loss of peripheral vision. It is typically caused by high eye pressure.

higher-order aberrations: Complex refractive errors or imperfections in the eye's corneal and lens focusing system involving many different areas of the cornea at the same time. Difficult to correct, these aberrations produce various symptoms including sparkles, ghosting, clarity, and problems with low light vision.

hyperopia: The medical term for farsightedness.

hypertropia: A condition in which the eye deviates upward. It is caused by a problem with eye muscles, or the nerves that control their actions.

hypotropia: A condition in which the eye deviates downward. It is caused by a problem with eye muscles, or the nerves that control their actions.

informed consent: A discussion between doctor and patient describing the alternatives to, and the potential benefits, dangers, and complications of a surgical or medical procedure the patient is considering. After all questions have been answered and an informed-consent document is signed, surgery or treatment can proceed.

intraocular lens: An artificial lens implanted into the eye to replace the natural crystalline lens. It is routinely used in cataract surgery but also used for other applications in which the lens has been identified as the source of visual deficiencies.

intrastromal corneal ring segment: Refractive eye surgery in which small arc-shaped segments of acrylic-like material are inserted in the body of the peripheral cornea. Their presence flattens the central cornea and treats mild forms of nearsightedness. They are marketed as Intacs in the United States.

irregular astigmatism: Astigmatism that cannot be corrected by simple eyeglasses. Its symptoms are vague and may include loss of contrast sensitivity. Simple LASIK surgery cannot correct it, but wave-front (custom) LASIK and rigid gas-permeable contact lenses often can.

iris: The pigmented membrane that surrounds the pupil. It contracts and expands in response to light level.

keratoconus: An abnormal thinning of the cornea that results in a cone shape producing very high astigmatism and nearsightedness. Gas-permeable lenses usually work well for a long time, but eventually a full corneal transplant may be needed.

laser: An energized source of light that has many applications in ophthalmology and other fields of medicine. It is used to reshape, destroy, or vaporize tissue and to slice precisely through tissue without affecting its surroundings.

LASIK: Laser *in situ* keratomileusis, a popular type of refractive eye surgery in which a blade is used to create a flap of tissue that includes epithelium and the middle layer of the cornea. Lifting the flap allows access to the middle layer of the cornea for reshaping by laser light energy.

LASEK: A variation of LASIK in which only the outermost surface of the cornea is lifted before laser application using toxic chemicals such as alcohol. This technique has been supplanted by a variant called Epi-LASIK, in which a blade is used instead of toxic chemicals.

lens: The normally transparent crystalline structure in the eye located between the anterior chamber and the vitreous. Together with the cornea, it bends light entering the eye to focus it, ideally, on the retina.

macula or macula lutea: The region of maximum visual acuity in the retina.

macular degeneration (age related): A disease of the central retina (responsible for central vision) that mostly occurs in people over 65 years of age. Although lost central vision cannot be corrected with eyeglasses, there are now effective treatments for certain types, including the injection of medications into the eye's vitreous.

macular hole: A defect or hole in the central part of the retina seen most often in older individuals.

myopia: The medical term for nearsightedness.

nearsightedness: A common visual condition which requires a person to be close to an object in order to see it clearly. It is caused by an image being focused in front of the retina, making distant objects appear blurred.

optic nerve: A thick bundle of individual nerve fibers that carries visual information from the retina to the brain

over-/under correction: A situation in which eyeglasses, contact lenses, or surgery fail to adequately correct near- or farsightedness because the correction they provide is either too weak or too strong.

pan retinal photocoagulation: Retinal laser surgery used to treat advanced diabetes and abnormal bleeding of the eye.

peripheral iridotomy/iridectomy: A laser, and sometimes a surgical procedure, that creates a small hole in the peripheral iris to treat or prevent closed-angle glaucoma.

phacoemulsification: A modern technique for treating cataracts by inserting microscopic probes into the eye. These probes use high-frequency sound waves to shatter the lens and suction the pieces out of the eye.

photorefractive keratotomy (PRK): An early type of refractive eye surgery that involves physically scraping away epithelial cells to allow access to the middle layer of the cornea so that it can be reshaped using a laser light.

posterior capsule opacity (PCO): A common consequence of cataract surgery in which a film develops behind the lens implant causing blurred or filmy vision. Vision is routinely cleared using a device called a YAG laser to vaporize the film. Commonly referred to as a "second cataract."

presbyopia: A natural consequence of aging in which the lens apparatus becomes less able to focus on nearby objects. It commonly starts in the late 30s to mid 40s and is treated by prescribing reading glasses. It should not be confused with farsightedness.

ptosis: A drooping eyelid.

punctal occlusion: A treatment for dry eye in which the tear drains in the eye are blocked either temporarily or permanently to increase the amount of tears in the eye.

pupil: The circular opening in the center of the iris.

refractive error: An inefficiency in the eye's ability to focus light on the retina. Examples of refractive errors are presbyopia, hyperopia, myopia, and astigmatism.

refractive eye surgery: Surgery to correct the need for glasses used for distance or near vision.

retina: A multilayered membrane that senses light entering the eye. It receives images focused by the cornea and lens, converts them into chemical and electrical signals, and transmits them via the optic nerve to the brain for visual processing.

sclera: The tough, dense, white outer covering of the eyeball. It covers all of the eyeball except the area enclosed by the cornea.

scleral buckle: A belt-like band applied to the sclera of the eyeball to surgically reattach a detached retina.

scotoma: A blind spot.

Sjögren's syndrome: A chronic, rheumatoid arthritis-like inflammatory condition of the tear and saliva glands that causes dry eyes and dry mouth. Often people complain of tooth cavities. Other organs in the body may be affected as well.

strabismus: A condition caused by the uncoordinated action of eye muscles resulting in eye misalignment. Depending on which eye muscles are involved, one or both eyes can turn abnormally in, out, up, down, or a combination of directions.

tarsorrhaphy: A rare medical procedure in which the eyelids are partially sewn shut to protect the eye from the effects of drying.

trabecular meshwork: A network of fibers located at the juncture of the iris, cornea, and sclera that is involved in the drainage of aqueous humor. When it is blocked, or fails to drain efficiently, the result is high eye pressure and glaucoma.

trabeculectomy: A surgical procedure for treating glaucoma in which a new filter is formed to release fluid and, thus, lower eye pressure.

trabeculoplasty: A surgical procedure for treating glaucoma in which laser energy is used to modify the eye's internal fluid-filtering apparatus to make it more efficiently filter fluid and, thus, lower eye pressure.

vascular endothelial growth factor (VEGF): A hormone that is secreted in the eye and other organs and tissues (including tumors) in response to a lack of nutrients and oxygen. The hormone induces the formation of new blood vessels which, unfortunately, are abnormal and fragile.

vitreous: A body of jelly-like material that fills the back portion of the eyeball. It presses the retina against the choroid, keeping the retina in place.

YAG laser: A specialized laser light machine used to treat glaucoma and posterior capsule opacity. The complete name is Nd:YAG (neodymium-doped yttrium aluminum garnet), which is a crystal used to generate the laser energy.

Index

Also Available from Sunrise River Press:

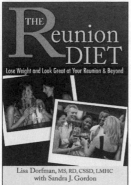
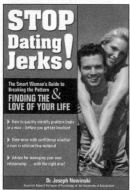
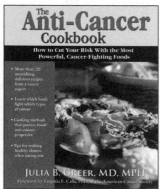